How to find health

Step 1
The origin of nutrition and vital functions.

Diego Pagani

ISBN-13: 978-1725674325

ISBN-10: 1725674327

English translation by Martina Bassi

DEDICATION
This book is dedicated to you.

I want to thank <u>Claudio Nicolig</u> for his fundamental support for the drafting of this text, without which the most scientific part would not have been so detailed and thorough.

Thanks also to <u>Lorenza Lullo</u> for introducing me to the world of food and for her help and support during the writing of the book.

Index

DISCLAMER

The author of this text is not a doctor, even if the information provided derives from medical scientific research. Diego Pagani is an independent researcher and with this book he does not intend to dispense, directly or indirectly, medical advice. The author can't prescribe a diet as a system of treatment for any disease, without the approval of a doctor. He only intends to offer health information to help the reader cooperate with his doctor in the common pursuit of well-being. In the case you use these information improperly, the publisher and the author assume no responsibility. Everyone is required to evaluate with common sense and wisdom the most appropriate curative and nutritional path. Each reader is free to evaluate all the necessary information contained in this text to compare the risks and benefits of the different diet regimens available.

1 ABOUT THE AUTHOR:
DIEGO PAGANI

I was born lucky; I had a happy childhood. I was loved and cared for in the best possible way by my parents, in addition to having the affection of all four grandparents. Aside from having had my tonsils out as a child, I have always had excellent health; to my great good fortune, I have never had to experience what it means to be really sick. During adolescence, my relationship with disease was non-existent. In consequence, I was not disturbed by the idea of sickness, and the idea even intrigued me a little. Over time, I experience the deaths one by one of my grandparents. Like any ordinary person, I have suffered a lot, but this, I thought, was normal. Like most people who have arrived at a certain age, I conceived of the emergence of diseases that lead to death as a natural consequence of life. How wrong I was!

Unfortunately, years later, my mother, who was just over forty, was hit by breast cancer, to which the "perfect modern medical science" opted for chemotherapy and removal of the breast. But as is so often the case with doctors, they could not save her life, but only lengthen it briefly. A few years after the operation, her breast cancer recurred in a more serious form, in the liver. Despite months of "cures" still based on chemotherapy, she died, after having first suffered terribly and been physically devastated. Nobody, but nobody, had warned my mother that proper diet could have saved her life. Today, in light of what I have learned, I am convinced that if my mother had changed her diet from the moment she was first diagnosed with breast cancer and later liver cancer, she would still be here and certainly would have helped me write this book.

Despite the death of my mother, my confidence in Western medicine was still unchanged and my ignorance on nutrition continued. I had not even remotely begun to suspect that such physical disruption could have been caused by unhealthy eating habits. Mistaken beliefs about nutrition can be passed down from mother to daughter with all good intentions, allowing a choice of foods that are apparently healthy, but in the long run, kill!

Apart from the family drama for me and my father, at the time I did not have any great curiosity in this terrible disease, not because it did not interest me as a result of killing my mother, but because I still had confidence in doctors and in "progress." Accordingly, both during the illness and after, I felt sure that the care and the methods applied had been the best possible, but, unfortunately, given the severity of the disease, it was impossible to do anything else.

A few years ago my father was diagnosed with throat cancer and underwent an operation. To my great thankfulness, he is now alive and has almost fully recovered. Also on this occasion, in addition to the sorrow one naturally feels at the illness of a loved one, I was not interested in the technical aspect of the disease because, once again, I assumed that the professional preparation of the doctors (favored by all these years of scientific research) was the only useful solution to help my father.

Sure, he smoked, and the onset of cancer was certainly encouraged by this undesirable habit, but now I realize that smoking was not the only cause and, probably, without that drawback, he could have healed without the need to undergo such a devastating surgery. While it is true that the operation saved him, but at the same time, it left him in a much debilitated condition, while leaving him in worse shape than before the surgery, plus brought him years of suffering that was certainly avoidable.

Today, in light of the information that I have since gained, I realize that if my father (in addition to giving up smoking) had changed his diet to one of good nutrition, his health might still be good. To some degree, I feel a little responsible for both the death of my mother and the great suffering that my father has experienced. Of course, I know I was not at fault for these events, but I realize that most of the information that I have collected over the last few years has in fact been available for many decades, perhaps more. This makes me think that if I had known sooner, I could have changed the course of events.

But this did not happen. Therefore, I hope with my books to help those who are still shrouded in the fog of ignorance and give you the means to find your way to thrive and especially to avoid seeing those you love fall ill needlessly and to undergo similar rounds of terrible suffering. In my first

40 years I never thought about my health, feeling myself to be normally healthy and in excellent health. Nutrition and especially its relationship with disease was not a topic of interest for me; I did not care about the topic and maybe I did not believe such a discussion was worthwhile, either. Left to my own devices, I was not particularly interested in various types of diets. I only knew the term "vegetarian" and I had never even heard the word "vegan." In my ignorance, the correlation between health and food was for me a completely unknown argument.

Until the age of forty years, I was nourished in the "traditional" way, namely eating a bit of everything—meat, fish, pasta, bread, rice, salads, fruit, etc. The only food that I never ate was cheese, not for dietary reasons, but just because I never liked it (thankfully). I have a normal physique, tending to slender. I am tall, at 1.80 meters and weighing 70 kilograms, and I've never been a big "glutton." I do not deny having spent evenings at restaurants enjoying the taste of some of my favorite foods, but I have always eaten just to eat; I ate just because "I needed to" take in nourishment. My relationship with food has definitely helped me change my eating habits toward the natural diet without having to regret my old eating habits; I repeat, I'm lucky.

In recent years, I have devoted my energy almost entirely to the study of nutrition and the effects it has on health. I have no medical training; I am not a doctor and I have not used expensive equipment. My only weapon has been a willingness to study and to gather information and collect many testimonies over the years from many people. Of course, I can speak from personal experience, because I have been able to carefully analyze the significant effects that a change has had on me, and on the people close to me. I consider myself a guinea pig, but a guinea pig lucky and happy to have discovered many truths!

I am convinced that, in this case, not being a doctor has helped me because I realized that too much knowledge (not always exact and often driven by economic interests) can easily create preconceptions. My initial ignorance allowed me to observe and experiment with my new frugivorous diet, observing events from a perspective completely absent from prejudice. My choice would appear to be unconscious and perhaps it was, but in addition to having perceived the sensation of being right, while I proceeded to what I was pursuing, my increasingly deepening studies assured me day after day that I was on the right path.

2 THE ORIGINS OF NUTRITION

One of the most dramatic biblical episodes is surely the expulsion of Adam and Eve from Earth's Paradise. The rabid God, throwing two poor innocents in the wild and uncoordinated nature, promising to one incredible labours and to the other atrocious pains in childbirth, is quite disturbing. A real misfortune for us descendants of such wretched ones. But, let's analyze the origins and structure of the myth. Meanwhile, we must say that stories like this are present in cultures far older than the Jewish / Christian one, and in each of these there is the dichotomy between the wonderful and simple life of the former and the degradation, the hunger and the pain of the later. The expulsion or the escape, are always consecutive to some terrible occurrence: a god disappointed and angry, or a cataclysm. Something, in short, makes man's life impossible and forces him to flee, to change his habits. Moreover, in all these myths it is clearly said that paradise, or shangrilla, as it is called, is on Earth. But where? Researchers and adventurers of all ages have been trying to find the Garden of Eden, no one has ever found it. Perhaps the problem is not geographic, but temporal. We hypothesize that the myth is much older than it has ever been believed. Shuffled by father to son orally, or indefinitely tied to the cellular memory itself, or even rooted in the most hidden meanders of the human unconscious, disguised in the loud crowd of our instincts. At this point we are catapulted in an ancient age, perhaps millions of years ago, a time when huge forests covered the valleys and plains of the central areas of the African continent, a time when our ancestors were just stretching their hands to seize a juicy fruit and bring it to the mouth. And archeology comes to us. Studies on the fossil remains of our ancient progenitors reveal us a lot. Certainly, somebody doesn't like the idea to descend from a being covered with hair, about a meter high, but those that until a few decades were just theories, are now widely demonstrated. Perhaps, we may have doubts about ancestral forces that have pushed or even push genetic mutations to change and evolve species, but the phylogenetic that rebuilds the human genealogy tree is now out of the question (see chart).

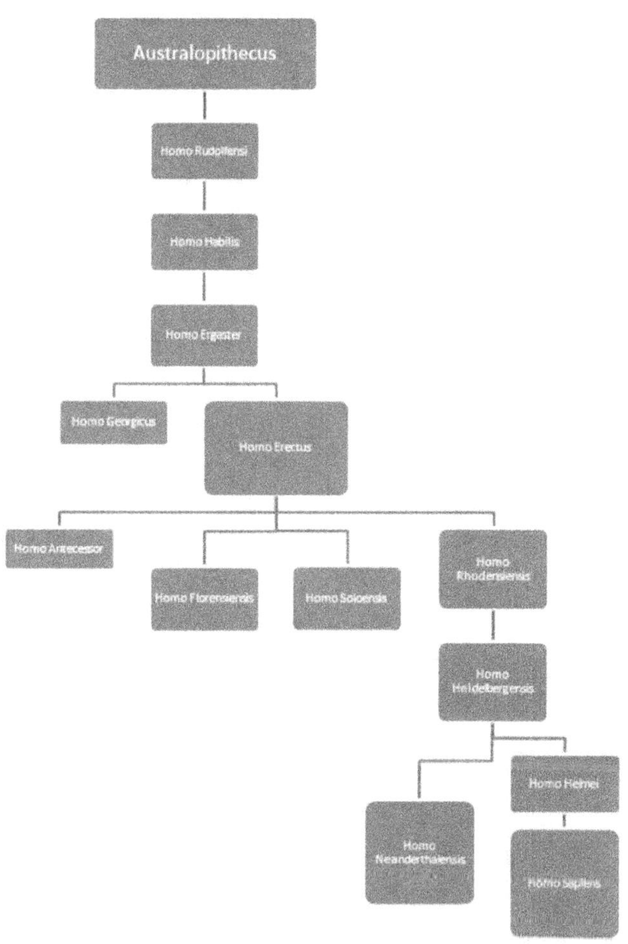

Australopithecus
Homo Rudolfensi
Homo Habilis
Homo Ergaster
Homo Georgicus
Homo Erectus
Homo Antecessor
Homo Floresiensis
Homo Soloensis
Homo Rhodensiensis
Homo Heidelbergensis
Homo Helmei
Homo Neanderthalensis
Homo Sapiens

In 1973, Donald Johanson discovered the remains of the body of an Australopithecus - from the Latin *australis*, "the south", and from the Greek *pitheco*, that is monkey, comprising parts of both legs, including an articulation, dating back 3.4 million years ago. In November of the same year, in Afar (Ethiopia), Yves Coppens, Donald Johanson, Maurice Taïeb and Tom Gray discovered the remains of a twenty-five-year-old adult female exemplar lived at least 3.2 million years ago. They called her Lucy, in honour of the Beatles song "Lucy in the Sky with Diamonds". She was 1.07 meters high, probably weighing between 29 and 45 kg, teeth similar to human ones, but still simian skull, with a skull capacity between 375 and 500 cm³; she was, however, a small specimen for its species. Subsequent findings show a marked sexual dimorphism, that is a large difference in size between male and female. The conformation of the skeleton parts gathered by the scholars shows that Lucy was perfectly suited to the biped locomotion, although it still led to a lifetime of arboreal locomotion. One may think that she would climb the trees to seek shelter from predators, to eat fruit or to spend the night. She's thought to have a social life and live in a group formed by adults and young. Her teeth were suitable for a diet based on vegetables harvesting and insects and lizards catching. Australopithecus had their heads with a flattened face, their frontal eyes allowed a stereoscopic vision, great to measure distances, to see hidden aggressors among the tall savannah herbs, but also to grab the branches of the trees on which they climbed and seized the fruit. Jaw and mandible beneath the skull, not protruding forward as in carnivores, are a sign of an adaptation to a frugal diet and to a semi-hard nourishment; this latter aspect is also shown by the very thick enamel layer, which makes the teeth hard and tough. This adaptation, with a slight decrease in the thickness of the enamel, has been preserved to the modern man. Their small incisors show that they were frugivores (in zoology is called a frugivore a living being that feeds mainly fruits or seeds) and folivores (a generic term that refers to all the animals that feed on leaves).

The reduction of canines is explained by some authors by the fact that the use of tools has rendered them useless as a means of threat (Darwin 1871, Simons 1972, Poirier 1973, Washburn & Ciochon 1974), according to others with the need to allow displacements side of the mandible in the "circular" mastication suitable for hard foods, fruits and vegetables (Jolly 1970, Dunbar 1976, 1983). The shape of the hand with the opposing thumb, other than that of anthropomorphic apes, indicates an adaptation to harvest seeds and fruits (Jolly 1970). The intestines had to be long enough, judging by reconstructions, as in animals that feed on plants. From Australopithecus, the family called Homo is born. They are our closest ancestors. The body with the passing of the eons stretches and straightens, the hair becomes more and more seldom, the size of the head and brain in it increases gradually.

The ability to walk erects is perfected, now they can afford to go deeper into the savannahs, abandoning tree protection. It improves the ability to build and handle tools and weapons, the first crafts, agriculture and early assemblies are born. In the time that flows, he colonizes both hemispheres, he becomes stationary and builds houses, villages. The past brings together the present, the modern man moves his footsteps on the ground, in fact the period ranging from the middle paleolithic of about 200,000 years ago to today sees the appearance and diversification of the Homo Sapiens species.

The precise dating of the first definable specimens *Sapiens*, traditionally placed about 130,000 years ago, has been moved by paleontological science back in time, around 195,000 years, from Ethiopian finds in volcanic tuffs of the Omo River valley. Archaeologists do not all agree on how long men exist as we know them, those who clean and well-shaved, perhaps dressed in a beautiful gown, we can meet without astonishing us in everyday life.

Some of the fossil remains of *Homo Sapiens Sapiens*, because this is the subspecies to which we belong, date back to about 113,000 years BC, but are incomplete and controversial to identify. We can say with some certainty that in the period from 50,000 years BC to the present day, men with our same size in all have begun to multiply and expand for the planet, leaving behind fossils and incontrovertibly human remains. The appearance and proliferation of modern humans occurs in a time of great climatic and geological changes, just during the last Earth's glaciation. In North America, the last glacial period is called Wisconsin Glaciation, because of rocky deposits studied in Wisconsin state in the United States and its beginning is set to 115,000 years ago. Since then, the ice cap advanced to the south, reaching the maximum extension around the 15,000 BC. This is a relatively long period, but something, perhaps a sudden climate change, led around the 13,000 BC to the dissolution of the entire ice layer within a few thousand years until the 8,000 BC when it was completely retreat.

The glacial period has been a worldwide phenomenon, affecting both hemispheres. Immense blanket of ice also formed in Asia, Australia and South America. In Europe, where it is called the Würm Glaciation, the ice layer extended from 70,000 years ago when it spread from Scandinavia and Scotland down to the UK, Denmark, Poland, Russia, Switzerland and Austria, as well as large portions of France and Northern Italy. The Würm Glaciation shared with Wisconsin the rapid and sudden dissolution, which always led around the 8,000 BC to the complete retreat of the ice.

The millennia during which the ice expanded has to have been very difficult and frightening for our ancestors, but the last seven thousand years of deglaciation must have been even worse. In fact, ice didn't dissolve in a homogeneous manner, but on top of the icepack, high at some points up to 3,000 meters, immense freshwater lakes formed. Millions and millions of liters of water kept from ever-weaker icy dams, which in their inevitable rupture flowed into the valleys of North America or Europe, giving rise to tremendous waves like Tsunami, affecting all the seas of the world. Seas and oceans, that during the maximum glaciation were about 120 meters lower than today, during the flooding phenomena climbed vertiginously without the waters retreat anymore. In addition, when the tremendous weight of that immense amount of water suddenly failed, the underground earth crust was projected upwards, giving rise to seismic waves of incredible and unimaginable intensity.

The Earth was all affected by terrible earthquakes, volcanoes resumed and Tsunami struck its shores. The increase in moisture caused by the volume of water released, bound to the ashes projected in the skies by the volcanism, contributing with the sun's darkening to the sudden fall in temperatures, led to the fall on the planet of heavy rains of frozen and muddy water. A true holocaust for our ancestors, who struck at irregular intervals, who tested their survival skills and perhaps brought the same human race close to extinction.

The Great Flood so vividly told in the Bible and in other 500 myths scattered around all the peoples of the world. Historical courses and appeals have characterized the existence of man and his ancestors in this long period of time. Periods where the forests stretched seamlessly for thousands of miles, ranging from great cataclysms, climatic changes, glaciations, which forced peoples to move or succumb, putting them in the face of drastic but necessary survival choices.

Because man from his distant origins was not and is not omnivorous, but forced to abandon a rigid diet of fruits and seeds by climatic and environmental conditions. As we have seen it is clearly deducted from its inherited physical characteristics almost unchanged by the progenitors: frontal eyes for stereoscopic vision, flat face with jaw and mandible placed under the skull, not able to rip flaps or interiors with the sunken face in the carcass of a dead prey.

The small teeth, incisive suitable for cutting the thin skin of a fruit; molars developed for long mastication of vegetable fibers; small canines, allowing easy circular movement for chewing. Teeth wear shows an abundance and orientation of microstries similar to those of predominantly vegetarian populations; it saliva with a pH between 6.5 and 7, so tendentially neutral, in contrast to the strongly acid of the carnivorous animals; the length of the digestive tract, a halfway between the very short of the carnivores, which allows a rapid transit of undigested flesh to avoid putrefactive phenomena within the organism, and the very long one of pure herbivores, characterized by the presence of pockets, to allow the slow absorption of vegetable fibers; a whole body graceful, not particularly fast, unsuitable to chase the prey; to finish a perfect, gentle hand, devoid of deadly claws, but with subtle fingers and opposing thumb, created to take, handle tools, create works of art and above all, to harvest delicate and juicy fruits from the plant that kindly give them. For those who still need some topic in the end, I have two amazingly convincing ones.

The study of human anatomy shows that, on the one hand, man has intestinal size, however inferior to those of a herbivore, on the other he has *taeniae*, *haustra* and semilunar folds like folivores! This is an adaptation present in many Primates, and in particular in all Cercopitecoidei (Old World Monkeys) and Ominoids [Hill 1967]. It consists in the fact that the longitudinal muscle layer is not disposed across the entire colon surface, but is limited to three parallel bands (*taeniae coli*). The contraction of these bands causes the remaining colon wall to protrude outwardly, so that the lumen extends outwardly into a set of three pockets (*haustra*). Such a constipation of the intestine slows down the transit of ingested foods, which is good for vegetable and fruit fibers, but is definitely deleterious in the case of meat and other animal tissues, which create putrefactive phenomena in persistent temperatures within the human body, resulting in the release of toxic substances such as putrescine, cadaverine and various dioxins, all highly carcinogenic substances.

The carnivorous intestines are very short and smooth, and in contrast to our basic, it has a remarkable acidity. This allows these animals to prevent the meat putrescence, demolish the protein faster and quickly remove the remains. Second point:

Unlike many species, including all carnivores, man is incapable of synthesizing an important enzyme, Urato Ossidase, most commonly known as Uricase, which plays a very important role in the metabolism of nitrogenous bases . These are the components of nucleic acids, including DNA and RNA, and present in large quantities in tissues.

The lack of enzyme Uricase causes our body to be unable to eliminate uric acid resulting from digestion of nitrogen bases. The acid accumulates in the blood and when organs such as the liver and kidneys lose their efficacy in time, it tends to crystallize in the synovial fluid of the joints. This fact leads to the swelling of the joints themselves to try to dilute the acid and to acute pains. It is then said that we took the gout. All this is well known, who doesn't know someone who doesn't complain of the swelling and painful crises that attach him to the joints of the ankles or feet? Perhaps what few know is that in our DNA the gene for the synthesis of Uricase enzyme exists, but is rendered inactive by some genetic mutations.

This is a truly ancient legacy of man, something that we carry from a distant past, perhaps before the primates, but for some reason we have decided not to use it anymore. Why? Lactic acid is a potent antioxidant, great for fighting free radicals and helping the body to protect itself against tumors and other diseases that they favor, so in low concentrations it is very useful. At this point, our ancestors are supposed to have favored a genetic mutation that, in view of a frugal diet and hard seeds, favor the free circulation of this acid by inactivating the enzyme specializing in its elimination. Unfortunately, evolution is a slow, actually very slow, phenomenon, and for the last 100,000 years, since man after the last glaciation had to turn the attention to meat and dairy products again, has not yet reactivated the above-mentioned gene. And he probably will not.

This is an important argument, because if man had been a carnivore, he would never give up such an enzyme as powerful and necessary for his health, risking, as it is now, jeopardizing the survival of the species itself.

A curiosity: 50% of human cancers hit the colon and has as its cause the meat-and-milk-based nutrition.

Every year the numbers increase, the mortality approaches 100%.

3 HUMAN BODY AND VITAL FUNCTIONS

The human body is a wonderfully complex machine. Ever since the first forms of life have made their appearance in the primordial oceans to date, evolution has tirelessly continued to improve and refine this fantastic instrument.

We have been forged to live healthy and happy, treading the surface of our beloved Earth to fully enjoy her fruits. Our greatest aspiration is to lead a life of joy and true vitality, full of enthusiasm, well-being, inexhaustible energy and endless taste for life.

But so it is not. Over time we turned away from the ideal. Illness has entered our lives. The society has swallowed us and with us also our health. Our vital energy is taken away from bad nutrition, pollution, stress and violence that surrounds us. Violence that we find in our own food.

To better understand what I'm talking about, to help you understand how to get out of this bad road, we need to know. Knowledge gives us the strength to react where ignorance keeps us in chains. Next pages of this book have this purpose. Unable to understand the basics of physiological nutrition, unless we first learn to know ourselves and the biological correlations that bind us to the environment in which we live.

4 ACID-BASE BALANCE

The pH is a simple measurement scale and immediate use that allows you to see the degree of acidity or basicity of any solution. The scale ranges from 1 to 14. pH 7 describes a state of neutrality, lower values measure acidity, values above basicity. The pH of human arterial blood has a normal range of between 7.35 and 7.45, so slightly basic. It is a very narrow range. Blood values less than 7.1 or above 7.6 are incompatible with chemical reactions occurring in our body, so with life itself. Lower values, in fact, trigger dramatic mechanisms, such as heart attack and cardiac arrest; Alkaline values above the range, however, lead to seizures and tetanic crises, when, for example, muscle strains begin to contract disorderly and in opposition to one another, causing paralysis and acute pain. In the extreme case this results in respiratory blockage and consequent death for asphyxia. The human body fights a continuous battle to keep pH within established limits, through cellular, lung and renal mechanisms, without counting the elimination through the skin.

The pH of the urine has a wider range, ranging from 4 in the sick, to 8 in infants. This last value is very interesting, as it certainly represents the optimum of iron health that we probably will not be able to reach again. For nine months, the infant lives immersed in amniotic fluid, which has a very basic pH in healthy mothers, equal to about 8.1, which gives us a clear indication of the degree of perfection of this value, given the importance for the nature of perfect development and total protection that the future born must have in the womb. It is spontaneous to ask at this point why the official pediatrics drives mothers to use pH 5.5 cleansers for baby hygiene and consider the use of basic detergents deleterious. Can it be hypothesized that the predisposition to allergies or other skin diseases can depend on this error? PH values in an adult's adult urine, below 5, reflect excessive work by the kidney, with the possible formation of acid calculations. The low frequency of pH in the urine may be a condition of body acidosis, a disequilibrium that causes tiredness, inflammatory conditions in the tissues and myelin of the nervous system, as well as an increase in free toxins and radicals that in turn cause other pathologies in a cascade process from nefarious results.

The causes of acidification can be numerous:

Taking of acidifying foods, such as animal proteins, milk and its derivatives, grains and refined sugars, legumes, tea, coffee, alcohol.

Mineral and vitamin deficiencies due to the ingestion of cooked, then denatured, foods or pharmaceutical synthesis supplements, which are therefore not organic and unassimilable by our body;

Contact with pollutants such as smoking cigarettes, SMOG, carbon monoxide, benzene, not least the notorious PM10 dust, etc.

Physical Overload: Muscle work involves an intense use of burned oxygen to produce energy, a mechanism called oxidative respiration or Krebs cycle, which, if too prolonged, and in the case where oxygen brought through the bloodstream is not enough to replace that consumed, it stops, replaced by energy supply from the least efficient glucose fermentation, which yields lactic acid as a metabolic waste product, which in turn accumulates in the tissues giving rise to cramps and precisely to the increase in blood acidity.

Reduced oxygen supply in sedentary or easy-to-take subjects of stress, anger and fear. The frequent, but rapid and shallow respiration characteristic of these situations, in fact, compromises the elimination of CO_2 from pulmonary blood resulting in acidification.

Abnormal disorders of excretory organs: kidneys participate predominantly in the control of non-volatile acids, and the skin, undervalued organ, eliminates every day a great deal of waste, toxic and acidic substances.

Use of drugs, synthesis substances, which usually put pressure on the kidneys and liver. Their side effects on these organs are deadly and under everyone's eyes.

At this point, it is clear how the balance between acidity and basicity within the body is one of the foundations of health. Every day millions of people go to hospitals or clinics around the world in pains or illnesses of all kinds. All these people have different symptoms, but the cause that has caused them to fall ill is always the same: acidification. All the acidic substances we enter into our body must be somewhat buffered or removed from the main organs. And this mortifies and debilitates the body, which uses all the resources it is capable of, and I assure you that there are so many, for this purpose. We can almost construct a chronological scale of what happens or happened in your body: first we are newborns, the intake of acidifying substances with nutrition does not cause us problems, heart, lungs, liver, kidneys and skin, everything is new and works in full efficiency, but right away, thanks to the loving attentions of our parents, certainly badly recommended, the powdered milk and the homogenized baby food put our organs really stressed out.

Then years pass, adding to the feeding meat, cereals and milk derivatives, the organs are still functioning, but some signs begin to warn those who hear, things are not going in the right direction, so the first allergies appear, illnesses like measles and chicken pox, considered normal among children, the first acne. The organs at some point begin to deteriorate. The efficiency of the lungs is compromised by a too sedentary life or perhaps by smoking because we don't want to miss anything. The liver and the kidneys lose efficiency in metabolizing toxic substances and eliminating them, maybe because we don't want to miss anything we've also exceeded in alcohol. The acidity level begins to increase. The concentrations of acids we enter into the body are higher than those we can eliminate. The body begins to accumulate and hide them somewhere everywhere, even to keep them away from vital organs. Fat deposits are born. Calcium is invoked by the arteries and bones to buffer the excess acids: arteriosclerosis and osteoporosis are beginning to be part of our life experiences. But let's continue. The deposits of acid substances increase again, the first wrinkles on the skin become dry and easy prey to mycoses and bacterial attacks.

The flesh we ingest produces uric acid crystallizes in the joints, the movements become slow, the back is curled. With old age the percentage of water in our body decreases and with it increases the difficulty of disposal of poisons.

What is missing? Oh yes. The death.

Maybe I was melodramatic, but this route has affected billions of people in recent man's history, and I have just described the story of a healthy individual. Because to born from sick and impure poisoned parents often leads the child to born already sick, already in the middle of the path. Moreover, I have not yet faced the tragedy of cancers and all the fatal diseases that are increasingly affecting humans.

Today's nutrition is made up of 90% by acidifying foods. They cause a continuous fatigue of the system, always under stress. Maybe it's the case of turning page.

Dr. Herbert M. Shelton, perhaps the most enlightened of American natural hygienists, once said, "*Blood should receive from the digestive tract water, amino acids, fatty acids, glycerin, monosaccharides, minerals and vitamins and not poisons. Unfortunately, our eating habits create poisons that poison the blood and the whole organism. Why? Because the bad approach of food in the same meal generates fermentation and rotting phenomena.*" This, which can be defined as a manifest of natural hygiene, denounces the risks of placing certain foods in the same meal.

Our cuisine combines food of all kinds in complex preparations, rich in spices and flavors, but mixing proteins with carbohydrates, for example, it slows down the intestinal passage. This increases the risk of putrefaction and the release of toxic and highly acidifying substances in our body. So attention is not only to what we eat, but how and with what.

Digestion products are commonly called *ashes*. There are alchemical foods like starches and proteins that release acid ash and acidic products, such as certain types of fruit, like citrus fruits, which instead cause alkaline ash. The acidic fruit, therefore, does not acidify, but alkalizes; also for the part that is not digested, just because it is sour, cleans the kidney ducts, subject to alkaline deposits.

Alkaline fruit, on the other hand, always gives rise to alkaline ash. It suggests that a fruit-based diet is always advisable.

Rich in organic substances and salts that can easily be assimilated to the body, it effectively combats the acidosis of the human body and is an impenetrable shield against the acid attacks that we are continually subjected to in our civilization.

4.1 What are acids and bases

The pure water chemical formula is very simple, H2O, two hydrogen atoms linked to an oxygen atom. Usually, however, in chemistry and above all in nature, there are no static situations and scientists always talk about dynamic equilibrium, that is constantly evolving and water is not an exception. Thus, a number of water molecules inside the solution will dissolve to form two ions, H + and OH-.

So we will have:

H2O ↔ H + + OH

Where the symbol ↔ indicates that the reaction takes place in both directions, then with a continuous transformation of water molecules into its ions and vice versa. In pure water the concentration of H + and OH- ions is exactly the same, so it is said that the solution is neutral.

Still in nature, however, it is difficult to encounter water free from any other content, there are, in fact, many substances dissolved, among which are very important acids and bases.

Acid is defined as any substance that, dissolved in water, free H+ ions, vice versa base is defined as a substance that in the same situation captures or better seizes H+ ions.

But how does this mechanism work? Maybe with a couple of examples we will be able to understand better.

One of the strongest acids in nature, and because of its danger we all know well, is hydrochloric acid, whose chemical formula is HCl, a chlorine atom bound to a hydrogen atom. Dissolved in pure water, it dissolves in its constituent ions, releasing H + and Cl-, according to the equation:

HCl Cl- + H+

Again, this is a dynamic equilibrium, hydrogen chloride molecules divide into the two ions and in turn many ions combine to form the same acid but, being this a very strong acid, the balance is shifted decisively towards the right of the equation, so the number of ions will be much higher than the number of molecules of the acid. We now assist in the release of many H+ ions and consequent acidification of water.

Another example: The strong base par excellence in nature is sodium hydroxide, well known by the name of caustic soda, commonly used to bleed the sink drains, the chemical formula of which is NaOH, a sodium atom bound to a oxygen atom in turn linked to one of hydrogen. When dissolved in aqueous solution, the molecule is divided into Na+ and OH- ions, according to the reaction:

NaOH Na+ + OH

It is, of course, understood another dynamic equilibrium which, being a strong base, is very moved to the right of the equation. The mechanism is similar to that of hydrochloric acid, but in this case there is a great release of OH-ions in the aqueous solution.

Why then the basic definition as "sequestering substance H+ ions"?As we have explained at the beginning of this brief dissertation, in pure water we find H+ ions resulting from the dissociation of the water itself and are precisely these to react with the excess of OH- released by the strong base according to the reaction: H+ + OH-H 2 O

Given the high concentration of OH-ions from the base dissociation, the reaction proceeds to the right, eliminating the vast majority of H + ions from the solution, hence the base definition. The aqueous solution becomes alkaline (basic).

Combining a strong acid with a strong base in solution gives rise to the salt precipitate:

HCl (Aq) + NaOH (Aq) NaCl (s) + H2 O

The symbol (Aq) means in aqueous solution, while (s) indicates solid state. It is interesting to note that the combination of two of the most reactive substances known in the art generates normal kitchen salt (sodium chloride).To combine a strong acid and a weak base solution, acidify the solution in part, since not all of the acid molecules bind to the base molecule giving its salt. Similarly, but speculating if we join a strong base to a weak acid, we will get a partially basic solution. This mechanism is the basis of all the acid-base reactions within our organism, where bases and acids of various types and different forces are constantly blended.

4.2 What is meant by pH?

In the previous paragraph we introduced the concepts of acid and base by putting them in relation to the concentration of H + ions present in a solution. Now it is necessary to give a measure, a scale that allows the easy use of these concentration values.

In 1909, Danish chemist Søren Sørensen introduced *Pondus Hidrogenii*, the potential of hydrogen or pH.

But what exactly is this number?

$pH = -\log10 [H +]$

PH is the negative logarithm based on ten of the concentration expressed in mole (atomic unit of measurement) per liter of H + ions in the free state in an aqueous solution. As we have said, in the pure water the concentrations of H + and OH are equal, for one liter of water both correspond to 1×10^{-7} moles, the pH will be $-\log10 [10^{-7}] = 7$. This is the pH of neutrality.

If H + ions (for acid addition or base subtraction) prevail in a solution, it will become acidic and its pH will drop to values ranging from less than 7 (weak acid) to 1 (strong acid).

On the contrary, the prevalence of OH-ions and the decrease of H + ions will lead to the basic (or alkaline) reaction of the solution, with a pH rise to values that will go from more than 7 (weak basc) to 14 (strong base).

4.3 Buffer systems

The pH of human arterial blood has a normal range of between 7.35 and 7.45. Maintaining pH between these values is of paramount importance, since variations beyond 7.1 and 7.6 are incompatible with life.

Red blood cells, for example, have a great plasticity, that means they are able to modify their shape so that they can pass through the narrowest capillaries, but their capacity decreases proportionally to the decrease in pH, that is the increase of acidity of the blood. At some point they will no longer be able to change their shape and enter into the narrower capillaries and whole areas of the body will no longer receive the right oxygen supply.

We will assist in the formation of thrombi and occlusions, which depending on the affected organ, will lead to severe pains to the necrosis of the organ, paralysis and death.

Within the human body one of the major sources of acid is the burning of glucose (with CO_2 and H_2O formation); moreover, cellular metabolism produces acids such as sulfuric acid, phosphoric acid, uric acid and lactic acid, metabolic processes, oxidation or degradation of various substances such as amino acids, phospholipids or carbohydrates and fatty acids. Acidification alters the arterial pH and must always be counterbalanced by "buffer systems" that act both at the cellular level and at the lungs and kidneys.

CO_2 produced during the respiration process is transformed inside red blood cells, thanks to Carbonic Anhydrase enzyme, in carbonic acid (H_2CO_3), which is immediately dissociated into bicarbonate ions (HCO_3-) and $H +$ ions. $H +$ ion is buffered by ossiemoglobin (with this term identifying hemoglobin during O2 transport), facilitating the release of the oxygen from the Hemes, which can thus spread to the tissues. The bicarbonate ion, which is the main vehicle for transporting CO2 into the blood, spreads from the red blood cell into the plasma.

At the level of lung alveoli, in the presence of large concentrations of oxygen and small concentrations of carbon dioxide, the opposite reactions occur. HCO3- ions fall into the red blood cells and bind with H + ions to form H2CO3 which in turn dissolves in CO2 and H2O, thus hemoglobin is again ready to receive oxygen. Carbon dioxide then spreads into the alveolus and is brought out of the body by lung breathing.

Summing up: Carbon dioxide produced at the cellular level becomes an acid in the blood plasma and at the pulmonary level, returned in the gaseous state, is eliminated with respiration. This process clearly shows us how by modifying the rhythm and volume of lung respiration we not only modify the oxygen supply in the blood, but also its acidity. Pathological obstruction of the respiratory tract or rapid but short-lived breathing, typical of stress or panic, are examples of factors that can lead to acidification of the blood.

Oriental people, through Yoga, have known for centuries how much breathing is important for maintaining good health.

The kidneys are the organs of the human body suitable for blood plasma filtration. Their task, however, is not limited to the simple extraction from plasma of waste materials, but it also involves the control and maintenance of many chemical equilibria, including acid-base. Each day, several liters of plasma cross the kidney and spread to a capillary level reaching the millions of tiny functional units, called *nephrons*, that are involved in filtering larger molecules and recovering from the filtrate the smaller molecules, still useful if not needed for the body. The nephron begins from the renal corpuscle, which, located near the cortical part of the kidney, the surface, is the actual filter. This then proceeds with the *proximal convoluted tubule*, with irregular shape, which, after some curves, moves towards the center of the organ and then continues to the bone marrow of the kidney with the Henle's loop, a U-curve, and return to cortical part with *distal convoluted tubule*, which finally flows into a collector duct leading the urine into the renal's pelvis. The nephrone has three functions. 1) Plasma ultrafiltration: plasma is filtered and only what is small passes filter meshes (catabolites, salts, H2O, etc.); instead the larger molecules remain in the capillary; this process takes place in the renal corpuscle. 2) Reabsorption of useful substances; the process takes place in the proximal convoluted tubule. 3) Concentration of the ultrafiltrated to form urine; the process takes place in distal convoluted tubule.

At this point it is easier to understand how the kidney can perform its control action on the acid-base balance. The bicarbonate ion, arriving at the nephron carried by the plasma, is able to pass the membrane of the kidney corpuscles, but it must be completely absorbed by the organ, to prevent the acidosis that would result from the newly production of carbonic acid. Resorption of the ion occurs through a process involving the Na + / H + pump located on the membrane that constitutes the wall of the proximal tubule. In practice, this pump enters H + ions in the tubule lumen, these bind to bicarbonate ions forming carbonic acid, which in turn, thanks to the presence of carbon anhydrase enzymes on the surface of the membrane that forms the tubule wall, is again converted into carbon anhydride and water. The anhydride is able to pass the membrane through diffusion, so it falls back into the tubular cell of cytoplasm, where thanks again to the anhydrase enzyme, this time cytoplasmic, returns carbonic acid and hence dissociates itself from hydrogen ions and bicarbonate ions. All this mechanism is necessary because the bicarbonate ion is not able to pass the cytoplasmic membrane directly, it must then be transformed into something else and then brought back to its original condition for reabsorption. Once again we are impressed by the wonderful complexity, but also the ingenuity of the human body. In the distal tubule of the nephron there are two other important reactions for the control of blood acidity. Both are involved in regeneration or new synthesis of bicarbonate and elimination of hydrogen ion through urine in the form of a titratable acid, such as H_3PO_4, or ammonia. The latter is the most efficient mechanism, which eliminates almost two-thirds of the non-volatile acids contained in the plasma.

4.4 Acidification of the organism

The wonderful acid-base blood balance control machine and consequently the human body works impeccably only if the individual is healthy, but also leads a healthy life and a healthy diet. It's not a game of words, but because of the complexity of the mechanism, variables that can compromise its functioning are so many. Food, sweetened drinks, smoking, drugs, stress, fatigue, and even too much sport, all these factors undermine our body's ability to maintain acidity within pre-established levels.

An example: gout. Have you ever wondered how this disease affects people at some point in their lives?

Purines are nitrogen bases found in nucleic acids. They are known to be nitrogenous bases of DNA and RNA, namely adenine and guanine, but purines are also xanthine, hypoxanthine, theobromine, theophylline, paraxanthine and uric acid.

The cells of the meat we eat are rich in purines, but man, like many close relatives primates and unlike many species, including all carnivores such as felines, is incapable of synthesizing an important enzyme, said Urate Oxidase, which can play a very important role in the metabolism of nitrogen bases.

In fact, purines coming from the diet are metabolized through various enzymes, such as Xanthin Oxidase, in uric acid, then in species provided with Uricase Enzyme, uric acid is in turn oxidized to 5-hydroxyisourate. The product of the reaction is unstable and turns spontaneously into *allantoin*, a molecule that represents the primary way of transporting nitrogen into the body. But we do not have the Uricase Enzyme. This means that the purine metabolism stops at the time of the synthesis of uric acid. This acid remains in the serum.

In the human genome there is a urine oxidase gene, rendered unfunctional by two mutations. Some scholars hypothesize that the loss of the enzyme has been an advantage for higher primates as uric acid is a potent antioxidant and protects against free radical attack, prolonging life expectancy and decreasing the incidence of cancers. The increase in uric acid in serum (hyperuricemia) leads to the lowering of pH values, thus the acidification of blood. The serum is saturated when the uric acid concentration reaches 7 mg per deciliter. Higher values pose the risk of precipitation of urate crystals (a salt), which are preferentially deposited in the articular capsules, and therefore acute gout attacks. The human body to counteract acidification frees uric acid through the kidneys, which are the biggest elimination pathway.

But let's take a step back. Purines are the nitrogen bases that make up nucleic acids, in layman's terms DNA and RNA. Not only the cells of the animals we eat are rich in nucleic acids but, of course, ours.

Every day millions of human cells end their life cycle and dying enter purines into the bloodstream, which are metabolized in uric acid. Perhaps, when scholars talk about the benefit of the absence of uricase enzyme for humans, they refer to the load of uric acid from apoptosis, that is, from programmed cell death. Surely, man has developed and evolved in the presence of low concentrations of endogenous uric acid, an excellent natural antioxidant in a fruit-based diet, tendentially rich in basic substances and poor of exogenous purines. But, as we all know, that diet has been abandoned and today man ingests large quantities of meats rich in purines daily, every day puts his kidneys under stress by forcing them into the hard task of eliminating large concentrations of uric acid.

Our bad habits do not stop there. Gout develops generally in the presence of obesity and excessive consumption of alcoholic beverages. In fact, obesity is associated with both an increased production of uric acid and a diminished elimination. Alcohol also reduces the renal elimination of uric acid and accentuates the catabolism of purines.Is not enough yet? Intensive use of drugs damages renal function. All this is added to the smoke, which with its poisons and decreased lung capacity contributes decisively to the acidification of the blood and puts the kidneys in crisis even more because of the big work they are submitting to them.

So comes the time when the machine starts to run badly. The kidneys begin to be suffering and the balance between acid and base crashes. The concentrations of uric acid rise to the precipitation point. Uric acid (Urate) salt crystals are formed in the joints and the pains become sharp.

At that point we will look in the mirror and observing a suffering and yellowish color face, we will tell us "old age has arrived".

5 THE IMMUNITY SYSTEM

Every day, every minute, every second, a terrible war is fought. The battlefield is one of the most extensive and complex in history. Used weapons, among the most advanced technologies ever developed. Chemical and biological weapons. It is an invisible war, but in the eyes of all of us and we are all struck by it, because it is for the salvation of our lives that is fought, it is in our bodies that the drama takes place.

It seems like the beginning of a '40s Political Sci Fi tale, right? Too dramatic?

We live on Earth's surface, immersed in a tiny atmosphere of gas that surrounds us, encircles us and penetrates us. And suspended in this atmosphere, billions of microorganisms live and multiply. With every breath we penetrate into our body. Some are innocuous, other friends; many of them deadly enemies.

No fear, man is an incredibly perfect, super-specialized machine. Do you know what is the best thing he can do? It is living on Earth. Obvious right? Millions of years of evolution have resulted in a body perfectly able to live and integrate with all the others present on the planet. At least until we try to sabotage ourselves, it will work fine.

The immune system is the set of organs specialized in fighting this war. Liver, spleen, lymph nodes, thymus, bone marrow, these are the generals who direct the battle, the white blood cells, the various classes, and the antibodies, the brave soldiers fighting it.

The capillary diffusion of the immune system and the number of organs involved, give an idea of the vastness and importance of the task to be performed.

White blood cells, called Lymphocytes, originate from stem cells within the bone marrow. Some cells are already specialized and are named Lymphocytes B, others remain undifferentiated until they reach the thyme, an organ just above the heart, where they are transformed into T lymphocytes (namely from thyme). Lymphocytes concentrate on lymph nodes and spleen, which should be considered as advanced control posts. The spleen, for the very high degree of blood spraying, is the organ that deals with the destruction of complexes formed by white blood cells and external antigens. Lymph nodes are spread throughout the body at the contact points between the blood flow and the lymphatic ducts; the latter collect the lymph which is a transparent yellowish liquid, ejected from the cells. Lymph nodes are real research stations and contact points with alien antigens. The most fitting example is the tonsils, which lie at the base of the larynx. They control the inhaled air during breathing, and the lymphocytes that are involved enter immediately into action at first contact with bacteria or viruses coming from the outside.

But what are antigens? Well, an efficient and fierce system like the immune system has the indispensable need to recognize a cell that is part of our organism from a bacterium or virus coming from the outside. Here, then, there are proteins on the surface of each cell, namely *antigens*, which, characteristics of each individual as fingerprints, allow identification as belonging to their own body, henceforth defined as *self-antigen*.

Bacteria and viruses also exhibit antigens, called *non-self*, on their bodies, and these are the ones that then give rise to the immune reaction. Antigens can be proteins present on the surfaces of microorganisms, but also pieces of protein chains that are free for our body, but we will discuss these later.

We try to reconstruct a possible chain of events: a number of bacteria enter through the respiration and given the irregular shape of the larynx, it slams against the surface of the tonsil. Here they come in contact with T-lymphocytes guardians. Our soldiers recognize antigens as non-self and immediately give the alarm. If the antigen is unknown, the reaction is slower. B-type Lymphocytes, among which we find white cells called *macrophages*, incorporate some bacteria and digest them; with a rather complicated mechanism the antigens present on these bacteria are collected and presented to the thymus, which stores the data and produces specific antibodies for that type. This takes time and obviously the bacteria in the meantime enter the body and begin to get to work. When the antibodies are finally ready, the real reaction starts. Antibodies are protein structures equipped with a specific antigen attack site, somewhat like the lock for its key. They are released in circles in massive doses and distributed throughout the body. When they reach the bacterium with the antigen for which they are constructed, they attack and wrap it completely. In this way, macrophages can recognize the enemy more effectively and attack it by force, destroying it.

The immune system is endowed with a kind of memory, traces every antigen encountered, and this causes the reaction to become lightning. This is a reason why, for example, measles can not infect a second time. After the first attack the defense becomes inexpugnable, we are vaccinated. The remains of the battle are then eliminated by spleen and liver.

Proteins are very active molecules in our body, so we cannot allow some chains of these circulate through the body without an apparent purpose, they can be the result of the destruction of bacteria or pieces of virus, or simply badly digested chains that, somehow, have been able to overcome the barrier formed by the walls of the digestive system. All these must be destroyed and it is the immune system that recognizing them as non-self antigen deals with cleaning.

This function of the immune system it is interesting to introduce a subject that is dear to me: *autoimmune diseases*. In an autoimmune disease, the immune system, for reasons not yet fully clarified, attacks self-antigens by considering them as enemies. That is, in a word, he recognizes like enemy cells that instead are part of the organism and attack them ruthlessly destroying them.

Graves' disease (hyperthyroidism), Rheumatoid arthritis, Tiroiditis (hypothyroidism), Vitiligo, Pernicious Anemia, Glomerulo-nephritis, Multiple Sclerosis, Type 1 Diabetes etc, etc.: autoimmune diseases affect millions people every year in the world and are countless, although ultimately they can be traced back to the same problem of the system: a pernicious attack of the organism against itself.

But what are the mechanisms that trigger the insurrection of the immune system?

And how does feeding fit in?

Molecular mimetism, this is the key that explains the birth of an autoimmune disease. Some microorganisms, such as bacteria or viruses, have on their surface identical antigens to those of the attacking organism.

The immune system starts the antibody reaction without being able to distinguish self from non-self and also attacks their cells. Here the mechanism is simplified to the maximum, because in reality the variables that come into play are many and varied. Normally, in fact, the immune system is perfectly capable of recognizing foreign antigens from their own and attacking only those that are actually dangerous. For some pathological reasons in some individuals this ability is lost and the "blinded" system indiscriminately attacks all the cells with that antigen.

Today, a correlation between feeding and autoimmune disease has been scientifically proven. Some proteins or parts of them, ingested with food, they can resist the attack of digestive juices and succeed, in the presence of pathologies of the digestive system, to overcome the barrier made by the walls of the stomach and intestine. Once in the blood circulatory system the immune system takes care to recognize and eliminate them with an antibody reaction similar to that practiced against bacteria or viruses. Some of these proteins have a shape and structure similar to those of the self antigens and therefore, we are once again faced with a case of molecular mimetism with all possible consequences.

Correlation between type 1 diabetes and cow's milk. This is an example of what we have written so far. The topic is serious and important that it can hit us indiscriminately in both the body and the affections.

In type 1 diabetes (not to be confused with type 2 diabetes, whose causes are closely related to the too rich Western diet), we witness the attack by the immune system against Pancreatic islets (also called islets of Langerhans, are tiny clusters of cells scattered throughout the pancreas). These cells, collected in globular formations, said islets, within the pancreas parenchyma, are suitable for production and release into the bloodstream of insulin hormone, to balance glucose concentration in the blood, in particular, with the function of lowering said concentration. Once the pancreatic islets are destroyed, the blood glucose rate splits upwards, out of control, causing serious damage to the body, with the only death result. The only weapon against type 1 diabetes available for general medicine is daily multi-dose insulin produced industrially by a few pharmaceutical laboratories.

Hygienist medicine proposes alternative forms of care that go beyond this discussion, but I strongly recommend the reader interested to give it a careful look. The results, though so harshly criticized by general medicine, are striking and unexpected, in some situations miraculous (though I do not believe in miracles, but in a proper and balanced care that has as its foundation a diet based on healthy and organic foods).

Let's return to the correlation between type 1 diabetes and cow's milk.

It is since 1992 that a Finnish laboratory published the results of a research on the incredibly high concentrations of *anti-albumin antibodies* in infants fed with cow's milk. Albumin is one of the major proteins contained in the cow's milk serum and often succeeds to overcome undigested the walls of the stomach. Unfortunately, albumin has, in its structure, protein chains similar to antigens present on islets of Langerhans. Here we closed the loop. The immune system develops anti-albumin antibodies and then - after a continuous war of years, as we continue to feed ourselves with cow's milk and its derivatives - it is no longer able to distinguish the enemy from the friend and the war becomes against us themselves.

According to the latest global statistics, the average age of the development of type 1 diabetes continues to fall; proved to be a genetic predisposition to the disease, the probability that our child if genetically predisposed present the disease is 50% in case of early weaning cows' milk.

Depending on the ingested animal protein, we may have antibody responses to different types of antigens, resulting in autoimmune attack on different organs. This is already happening, judging by the amount of existing autoimmune diseases and the number of people affected every year.

In conclusion: a healthy, well-fed body will be perfectly capable of keeping the attacks of pathogenic microorganisms at purely unconscious levels, we would not even notice it being in progress.

Man did not evolve on earth to be sick.

Continuous intake of foods of animal origin, chemicals, preservatives, dyes, and so on, chemical, mechanical and psychological environmental pollution... All of these causes an imbalance in the body, limiting the functionality of our organs and systems. It is a continuous and inexorable drift towards the disease, whatever it is.

How much longer we'll ignore it and continue to move forward in that way?

6 THE ENZYMES

In order for two or more molecules or atoms react with each other, it is necessary that collide at the right speed and in the correct position.

Increasing energy in the form of heat corresponds to an increase in the motility of the molecules and hence an increase in the number of clashes. Reactions are facilitated. The energy that I have to enter into the system to initiate the reaction is said *activation energy*. In the case of endothermic reactions, that is without release but with energy consumption, I will have to continue to provide energy for the reactions to continue until the reagents are exhausted.

Instead, in the case of exothermic reactions with the release of energy, the process is self-sustaining until exhaustion. It is important to emphasize that, if no energy is added, many chemical reactions do not occur, or, at ambient temperatures, occur at an insufficient speed for our purposes. There is, however, a way to lower the value of activation energy: through the use of catalysts. The catalyst is a medium that facilitates and accelerates chemical reactions without being consumed or modified. In other words, it provides a support, said *attachment site*, to approach and put in the right position the reagents molecules. In this way they find themselves in the best position to react. Substantially, the catalyst lowers the activation energy or better the temperature necessary for the reaction to take place.

The catalysts are reversible, that is they can favor both reactions in which one or more reagents are combined to form a product, or the opposite, where a molecule is disrupted in simpler molecules.

The catalysts are very common in nature and are both *inorganic* (an example is the platinum catalyst of car mufflers, which makes it easy to eliminate the toxic compounds resulting from the combustion of hydrocarbons), both *organic*, such as enzymes.

At this point we can define enzymes as complex proteins that act as catalysts in chemical and metabolic reactions in our organisms, or best, in all living organisms on planet earth. Without them, life could not exist even in its simplest forms.

To better understand the importance of enzymes, one must really understand that they are involved in all, really all chemical reactions of our organism. It is thanks to an enzyme, DNA-polymerase, that DNA is duplicated when the cell is divided into two daughters. RNA polymerase, on the other hand, reads DNA by building a pair of homologous RNA bases that will then be carried by the cell nucleus into ribosomes for protein synthesis. Only these two examples give the idea of how much enzymes are important. Energy production, immune defense, transport of information, protein synthesis, fatty acids, vitamins and anything else, digestion, elimination of toxic substances, etc., etc., no enzymes would work anymore, even the mechanism of memory or thought itself.

It is thanks to the enzymes if the average temperature of our body only attests to 98.6°F (37°C), otherwise it should be much higher for metabolic reactions to take place, with adverse consequences on the stability of the chemical structures that participate in our physiology, certainly not very compatible with the life.

In all this, a class of enzymes is particularly interesting for our discussion: the *digestive enzymes*. This class of enzymes are involved in the digestive process in our digestive system. They are found in saliva and gastric juices and intervene to facilitate the degradation of the food and to make possible the absorption of nutrients by the walls of the stomach and intestines. Among these we find *lipase*, which intervenes on lipids, *amylase*, on carbohydrates and *proteases*, on proteins.

Digestive enzymes are present in raw foods. Especially in fruits and vegetables.

Even in meat (if raw), but in relatively small concentrations. The presence of this enzymatic class in foods greatly facilitates their digestion by our body, it can be said that these foods digest themselves. Unfortunately digestive enzymes are very delicate. Like many proteins, they are thermolabile and undergo transformations during cooking that inhibit their functioning. Even traditional chemical or mechanical preservation methods compromise its operation: in the end it is for this reason that cooked or processed foods last longer. For those who eat essentially cooked or preserved food, the need of replacing or integrating lost enzymes arises with those produced by our body, in particular from the pancreas, the liver and the stomach wall and poured into the lumen digestive tract through the gastric juices. This causes a big work on the organs mentioned above, with great energy expenditure.

According to recent studies, it seems that the eating habits of cooked foods have led the human pancreas to be hypertrophic, reaching, in relation to body size, two to three times the size of the same organ in the species closest to us. If we think that the type 1 diabetes is linked to a dysfunction of the pancreatic islets of Langerhans, who knows that there is a correlation?

It is evident that a raw food vegetarian diet ensures the necessary enzyme intake for a proper and non-tiring digestion. However, even if you still do not feel ready to abandon the cooking of food, it would still be good during the meal, ingesting a sufficient amount of raw vegetables to help and sustain the work of our body.

7 THE LIVER

Many of us had their first experience with alcohol at a young age. A glass of wine with friends or during a family toast, the occasions are innumerable and varied.

This is a good starting point to begin talking about one of the most important organs of the human body: the liver.

The portal venous system collects blood from the intestinal wall and spleen and delivers it directly into the liver.

When we ingest a food or drink a glass of wine, the digestive system assumes the task to disassemble it and break it up into its basic primary components and then, through the absorption of its walls, make sure that the nutrients arrive at blood, conveyed through the portal vein directly to the liver. I said nutrients, but it's also what happens to the poisons, toxic substances and drugs in general. All this is closely related to one of the many function of this organ, the control and elimination of toxins from the blood. The obligatory pathway that is to deal with all the ingested substances is known in pharmacology as the "first-pass effect" and as you may already imagine it has consequences that greatly interest the pharmacists.

The liver is the first bastion which stand up to defend our body from all those substances which, for various reasons, are recognized as enemies or toxic. Among these there are certainly drugs. This is one reason why the tablets we ingest have concentrations of active ingredient tens if not hundreds of times more than necessary: due to the first-pass effect the drug just entered our body meets the liver and these, recognizing it for what it is, a poison, try by all means to destroy it. Only a small portion is saved and can reach the blood and through this its target organs.

Here we begin to understand why strict requirements appear in the leaflets of all medicines on its ability to damage the liver.

But let's go back to our first glass of wine. Of course all the steps that will follow are simplified to the maximum, this book is certainly not the place for a thorough discussion of physiology.

The alcohol content in wine is rapidly absorbed by the walls of the stomach, enters into the capillaries that form a dense network around the digestive tract and through them into the portal vein that conveys it within the liver, which is also sprayed by a dense network of capillaries. Thus, the liver enters into contact for the first time with a massive dose of alcohol, recognizes it as a substance to be deleted and is activated to metabolize, that is splitting its molecules to make it harmless. This first contact finds our liver unprepared, the efficiency with which it attacks the alcohol is not very high, the organ still needs to find the most effective system for elimination. A good alcohol concentration at this point is able to go undisturbed and enter the blood stream. With this it reaches the brain, which will be affected by his first hangover.

How many of us, speaking of *memory*, go immediately with the mind to the ability of the brain to remember the salient events of our lives? The truth is that the human body in its complexity has other less known storage mechanisms. The immune system, for example, remembers viruses and bacteria against which it has fought, and this greatly accelerates its ability to respond in case of relapse: this is the reason why you get measles only once in your life.

So also the liver is able to integrate into its capabilities the best procedure for the elimination of a substance in order to be faster and more efficient. Here is why we continue to make use of liquors, our body always perceives the lesser of the harmful effects, and we can boast with friends that we can drink without getting drunk! But it's not all gold that glitters. A boy's liver is young, healthy. Its ability to metabolize substances is at maximum efficiency. How long can we hope to continue without causing him irreversible damage?

In fact, it is a chronic drunk feature getting drunk with the first glass: this is due to the inability of the liver, now seriously ill, to eliminate even the smallest amount of alcohol that ends up circulating. This is the much feared, common liver cirrhosis.

It is a curve that can easily be represented graphically: at first the liver is slow in the metabolisation of alcohol, then the memory comes into play and its efficiency increases enormously, then the continuous poisoning takes over and with it the inability to metabolize. Unless you find a healthy and unlucky donor, at this point there is only death.

But let us pause for a moment on the memory mechanism. This works for all the substances with which the liver comes into contact, including the drugs.

A striking example is its continuous fall of efficiency of sleeping pills or tranquilizers in general. In fact, in addition to very complex mechanisms that come into play at cellular receptors, the best liver elimination capacity forces the patient to slowly increase doses. This allows him to continue to take advantage of what he thinks to be the benefits of cure, but on the other hand he brings him daily closer to the poison level.

There are no longer any doubts about the adverse effects that bad drug use may have on the liver.

First pass effect and memory. Here are two capabilities of this incredible organ, but the liver still has many secrets to reveal.

What is the liver ultimately? A gland: the largest gland in human body.

The liver receives blood from the whole organism and through a complex system of mechanical and metabolic reactions it purifies it: not only from the substances we ingest but also from the refuse products of our organism, among which to make examples are the remains of red blood cells that have terminated their life cycle, viruses and bacteria inactivated from the immune system, molecules or parts of them result of metabolic processes, etc. All this is meticulously disassembled in its basic components; what's needed go back in the circle, while what is not needed is collected in the bile and through the bile ducts, stored in the gallbladder. From here it will be poured into the intestinal lumen to contribute to digestion of fatty acids and then eliminated with the stools.

Here is the macroscopic function of the gland, bile production.

The bile is a bitter yellowish-greenish liquid with a remarkably basic pH. Its function is of great importance, in fact, it must counteract the effusion of acids from the stomach to allow the intestinal enzymes to crush the large lipid chains, reducing them to small particles that can overcome the intestinal walls. This allows the digestion of fat, oils and Fat-soluble vitamins such as A, D, E and K. It is at this level that we assist in the transformation of Beta-carotene into free A vitamin. The bile also has an antibacterial function and promotes intestinal peristaltic movements, thanks to which the feces are pushed toward the last intestinal tract for elimination. The liver helps control the concentration of glucose in the blood. In fact, in it occur *gluconeogenesis*, glucose synthesis from amino acids, lactic acid and glycerol, *glycogenolysis*, glucose synthesis from glycogen, *glycogen synthesis*, a mechanism contrary to the former that produces glycogen from glucose, and finally deals with the demolition of insulin. The glycogenolysis is stimulated by the hormone glucagon, synthesized in pancreatic islets with insulin, in order to counter the fall in the blood sugar level from this stimulated.

Not everyone knows that the brain obtains the energy it needs solely and exclusively through the Krebs cycle or glucose oxidation. It is in simple words the combustion of glucose with oxygen to produce the necessary calories. Glucose is therefore a highly effective fuel, the only one capable of satisfying the intense brain activity, and explains why low blood glucose concentrations generate tiredness, apathy, low concentration threshold and severe headaches.

High concentrations of glucose, on the other hand, are the cause of body poisoning, as can be easily deduced from the major problems people with diabetes suffer. The arteries lose elasticity, blood pressure increases and also the work of the heart, wounds work hard to heal, bleedings increase and so on. It's a delicate balance, glucose starvation of our body, its toxicity. The blood glucose rate, therefore, has a very high importance and its value must be very precise with minimal variations and rests on two delicate pillars synthesized in the pancreatic islets of Langerhans, insulin and glucagon, which perform their action through the liver.

The importance of these two organs is blatant. The liver is also the home of the synthesis and storage of fatty acids.

Fats that a noisy and careless press turned into a fetish, the number one enemy, the evil of the world and in the venom that will take us all to extinction. The reality is different. As with everything related to the complexity of this incredible machine that is the human body, it is always in a harmonious way to manage the balance, the simple balance.

Lipids, the most correct and precise denomination, are a necessary brick for life. The cell membranes of all plant and animal life forms have a lipidic structure. This means that without them there would not exist life on the planet! Many vitamins and hormones have a lipid-based structure. Lipids are a reservoir of energy that our body builds up and then use as needed. The lipid layer on our body plays a key role in its thermal control. The hydrolipidic layer covering our skin has the very important function of defending it and making it waterproof to the attacks of chemical and biological pathogens. And yet a thousand things that would be hard and perhaps boring to deal here.

Does anyone still have any doubts about the importance of lipids?

But then triglycerides? Cholesterol?

Equilibrium.

In this book we are dealing with the benefits of a diet based only on fruit.

A diet without heavy saturated animal fats. Do you think that because of a similar diet we will assist in body disruption or on the outbreak of cell membranes? No!

Thanks again to our liver. It is in fact the home of vital biological mechanisms for life, such as the synthesis of fatty acids: yes, gentlemen! Including triglycerides and cholesterol. A healthy liver and a proper diet will guarantee the respect of the ecological balance and healthy living.

Continuing to bomb the human body of animal foods compromises that balance. An incredible amount of lipid from digestion flows into the lymph nodes adjacent to the intestine and then from these into the bloodstream and from here it reaches the liver. Part of this sea of fat reaches the body points where it is needed, one part will be stored in special fat cells for future needs and a large part of it will necessarily be converted or destroyed by the liver itself. As for alcohol, how long can last all this? At some point efficiency in elimination is compromised. Cholesterol and triglycerides are poured into large amounts in the blood and get stuck to the vascular walls, and the liver itself becomes a lipid deposit (fat liver), dramatically losing its functional capabilities. The fat cells continue to reproduce and grow in numbers until it covers the entire body and to bring us into pitiful overweight and obese individuals who barely manage to accomplish the basic movements.

A curiosity that may affect: there is a correlation between number of fat cells and hunger. They are tanks with the sole purpose of storing lipids. During the weight gain phase they are created and filled. Now we hypothesize we want to lose weight. Finally we look in the mirror and see the state in which we are reduced, we decide to give us a set and lose weight. Here is an unexpected enemy coming to our horizon. During the weight loss phase, the fat cells are emptied, but not eliminated. They continue to live on the basis of their assigned cycle, but throughout the time they continue to ask for being filled, screaming, emit hormones that excite hunger sensors and make our diets a real war.

This is one of the reasons why taking back weight after a diet is so easy.

This is one of the reasons to keep our kids in shape and lean; if they begin to accumulate fat at a young age then it will be difficult for them to lose it.

At this point it is urgent a small summary: bile production, filtration and elimination of toxins, control of blood sugar levels, synthesis and control of blood lipid concentrations, removal of dead cells with recovery of useful substances, all of this is the liver.

The ingestion of fats, sugars and alcohols, industrial chemicals, preservatives and colorants, hydrogenated fatty acids, solvents, and so on, puts stress on this organ every hour, every day.

For those who had not yet thought of: the function of elimination of toxins regards all those that circulate in the body through blood, not only those who come through the digestive system.

That is why even for smokers, the cargo load from cigarettes will not only damage the lungs, but because of the very high absorption capacity of the finest and delicate membranes of the pulmonary arteries, it will find the way to the blood bed, reaching all the organs and charging the liver of a new job he certainly does not need. Here is how the incidence of liver disease for smokers and drinkers increases in a quadratic manner, not corresponding to the sum of the two ills, but to their multiplication with disastrous and catastrophic effects, not only at the human level.

Think of family drama, but also economic, if we focus on the costs that these diseases have on society, even at the expense of patients morally more deserving of care.

And again, with the same mechanism we can understand the nefarious damage to the liver that chemicals we breathe through the polluted atmosphere in which we are perpetually immersed.

As the liver gets tired, his functions fail. Balance is compromised. Not destroyed toxins are poured into the blood and the human body has to look for new ways to eliminate it. The kidneys and the skin are natural pathways. We are now seeing an increase in the number of diseases of these two organs, dermatitis, acne, kidney stones and many more. If we were to get hold of the statistical tables that the Ministry of Health periodically receives on their desks, we could easily see how many are the numbers we're talking about. The population becomes more and more ill and for those who want to see reality without preconceptions or, worse, without wanting to defend economic interests of sorts, true motivations are obvious.

But do not demoralise more than we owe. The chance to get out of this vicious circle exists and it's just our beautiful body to show us the way. In fact, the liver, with all its load of functions, is an organ with a very efficient ability to regenerate. It takes five months to a year to see it almost reborn and return to its normal activity. Its regeneration capacity is so high that, if we take a part, it is able to grow again. This is the mechanism that allows liver transplants even among living people. The section removed from a compatible person has high chance to take root in the new host organism giving him again a new life. Attention, this should not be an excuse to devote ourselves to the destruction of our liver ...

It becomes clear as you embark on a virtuous diet that it can greatly improve your lives. In a few months the organ, though obviously not too compromised, will again perform its normal functions and life will return to smile.

I am often asked how health can be compatible with a fruit-based diet which ultimately is full of sugars (fructose, glucose and various starches) and poor in fat, those of animal origin entirely absent. The answer to these questions is hidden between the lines of this chapter. To begin with, it should be clarified that sugars are not present in all fruits in the same concentrations. Some fruits are rich, others poor: vegetable fruits, such as zucchini, pumpkin, peppers, cucumbers, tomatoes, eggplant, have very low concentrations of glucose and fructose.

So a varied diet, which spaces between the incredible choice of different fruits, will already be well balanced. Some scientists believe that the fruit of the apple, being characteristic of the original places of man and probably the primary fruit of the original diet, well represents with its composition the right equilibrium of the nutrients we need. At this point it should be emphasized that a fruit-only diet does not add toxins to our body, which is therefore able to function at its best.

Liver and pancreas succeed through the mechanisms we have already discussed to better control the concentration of glucose in the blood. The ingested sugars are converted completely into glucose. Then this, depending on our body's needs, undergoes other transformations in fatty acids or proteins themselves. Because if it is true that with the fruit we ingest many sugars, it is also true that we **do not** assimilate fatty acids of animal origin.

It is the liver who deals at this point to overcome this lack of food by synthesizing the fat that our body needs in the dose and in the perfect quantity. So the apparent sugar surplus ultimately proves not to be such. Everything is used without waste or excess.

8 THE DIGESTION

Petroleum is a dense, oily liquid of very dark color and nauseous odor. Have you ever thought of putting it directly into a car fuel tank? Well, the result, as we can easily imagine, would be the death of the engine and several hours of labor in the garage to clean up the organ from all that black mud. The point is that the engine in order to function properly needs the right fuel. Oil has to be refined and undergo several chemical transformations to become gasoline and do not damage our engine. So it is also for the human body. Food, in its natural state, must be altered to become fuel for a living organism. Unlike cars, fortunately for us, the biochemical center able to make all the necessary mechanical and chemical transformations, is an integral part of our own body, the digestive system.

We will now enter the chain of events leading to the digestive process.

Human teeth have different shapes based on the effect they have on food during mastication, cutting, crushing, breaking and grinding, all to reduce the bite in small parts, which, thanks to the movements of the tongue, are mixed with saliva secreted from the glands in the oral cavity. It is a transparent liquid composed of 99.5% water and the remaining 0.5% by enzymes that begin a first digestive phase. These are the α salivary amylase, an enzyme that at pH 7 starts the demolition of carbohydrates, and salivary lipase, which instead, deals with the first demolition of lipids. This first phase is very underestimated. Our society imposes increasingly frenetic pace and the time dedicated to the meal becomes shorter. In addition to reducing the quality of ingested food, chewing becomes quick and hasty, the bite swallowed almost whole. This compromises the subsequent stages of digestion, making it longer and more laborious. It is important to know that acidity of lipase lasts for a long time and continues its lipid scavenging effect even in the stomach, up to the intestine, where the intestinal lipase comes to its aid. It is evident that a good chewing allows the best digestion of lipids.

At this point the bite takes the name of *food bolus* and it's swallowed. It crosses the larynx and is conveyed to the esophagus. It is a tube of soft and elastic tissue, equipped with a smooth muscle arranged in annular manner around it. The organ runs down, crosses the diaphragm to end in the stomach. Its characteristic musculature exercises those that are called *peristaltic movements*, which with their sinusoidal pace guarantee the passage of food even if we were to head down.

A curiosity: the hiccup is due to a lack of synchronization between the respiratory movement of the diaphragm and esophagus movements, the unharmonious of these two movements causes the so annoying hiccup: fortunately holding his breath for a few seconds it allows the two organs to regain synchronism and everything is resolved.

The bolus descent continues with the crossing of the cardia, the sphincter that closes superiorly the stomach to prevent the rise of gastric juices into the esophagus, which, alas, not always able to do. The problem of acid reflux affects every year an increasing percentage of the population.

We are now in the stomach, a volume of about a liter, wrapped in a thick smooth muscle that with its movements contributes to its content shuffling.

The mucous membrane that lines the walls of the stomach presents numerous *microvillus*, which greatly increase the surface area, interspersed with glands that secrete gastric juice, almost 500 ml *pro die*, composed in turn by enzymes, mucus and hydrochloric acid.

The acid performs many tasks: it eliminates the bacteria present in the bolus, dissolves the cementitious substance that keeps the cells of food together, destroying it, and finally activates the *pepsinogen enzyme*, transforming it into pepsin, acting on peptide bonds of proteins, breaking their amino acid chains.

The function of mucus produced at the mucous level is precisely to defend it from the attack of pepsin. Without it gastric juices would digest the same walls of the stomach. Even in this case, in the presence of various pathological factors, we can observe the lack of efficiency of the protective system, then we speak of peptic ulcer, a form of very painful mucosa inflammation, which in case of perforation of the wall quickly leads to death.

As we have seen, the stomach generally has a function of dissolution and digestion of proteins; its absorption capacity is minimal and limited to a few substances such as water, vitamins, glucose and alcohol. This is one of the reasons why the action of these substances is so immediate.

By now the reader will understand that I love to share my explanations of various news and curiosity. Do not hold it against me, but I am convinced that my old habit can break a bit the monotony of an otherwise boring subjects. Here's a gem:

In the fifth century BC, Hippocrates, the father of modern medicine, described a remedy composed of a bitter powder extracted from the willow bark, to calm the pains and lower the fevers. Medical literature, however, refers to even more ancient news, already the Sumerians, the ancient Egyptians and Assyrians talked about it, and the remedy was even known by American Indians, and this suggests that it is truly ancient.

The active ingredient in the willow bark extract was isolated in 1828, but in 1897, history takes an interesting bend when Felix Hoffmann succeeded in attacking an acetyl group to what until that day was salicylic acid, transforming it into acetyl-salicylic acid, the same benefits, minor contraindications. That chemist worked for Bayer and had just synthesized *aspirin*.

Now I come to the point. Aspirin is definitely the pharmaceutical drug most sold in the world, even long-lived, and one of the few to be able to be absorbed quickly by the stomach lining. The problem is that it is a rather aggressive acid. Although, in recent commercial declarations, it has been buffered in some way, its side effects are quite persistent. In addition to acidic action directed at the gastric mucosa, it has a suppressive action against the synthesis of the protective substances of the wall itself. Another effect, considered positive in some heart therapies, is that of anticoagulant. But all this makes it quite dangerous, as ulcerative and hemorrhagic agent.

But let's get back to digestion. The contents of the stomach when it is ready to pass into the intestine has become a milky and acidic mass that takes the name of *chyme*.

The small intestine is divided into three main sections: *duodenum, jejunum* and *ileum*. Once in the duodenum the chyme is sprayed with the bile produced by the liver. This brings the pH to about 7 and emulsifies lipids to allow lipase enzymes to disintegrate them more easily. The absorption action, proper to this organ, is mainly carried out in jejunum and ileum tracts. To increase the absorption surface enormously, the intestinal walls exhibit numerous *folds* or patches, whose mucous membrane has protuberances, called *villus*, of about one millimeter long, about 3000 per square centimeters (465 Square Inches).

Cells that coat the villus have in turn hundreds of reliefs called microvillus. Thanks to the circular folds, the absorbent surface of the intestine has increased by 3 times; the villus lead to a further increase of this surface by 10 times; the microvillus of another 20 times. Thus the intestinal surface available for absorption is about 300/400 square meters (4,305 Square Feet).

Within each villus runs a blood capillary in which the nutrients are poured, mainly glucose, amino acids, salts and vitamins. At this point, the absorption of many drugs or poisons is also taking place. Everything is conveyed to the *portal system* (it is a portal system when veins coming from a capillary bed are subdivided a second time, in other capillaries) and from here it quickly reaches the liver, which will take care of their metabolism.

Regarding fats, the absorption mechanism is more complex. This is due to the fact that they are hydrophobic, that is, they are not water-soluble. This is something that we can easily check in the kitchen. If we put oil in a basin, it tends to float because of its low density, but above all it tends to blend into bubbles, said *micelles*, in order to reduce as much as possible the surface contacting the water. Under these conditions, its transport through the blood is impossible.

The short-chain fatty acid are completely hydrolyzed by pancreatic lipase enzymes, they are therefore able to pass by diffusion the mucosa of the villus and, once in the bloodstream, follow the same path of other substances to the liver. About complex long chain molecules, the way to go is different. Once emulsified and reduced to simple chains, fatty acids pass through diffusion the cell membrane. Once in the cells of the intestinal mucous membranes of jejunum and ileum, with considerable use of energy, they are reassembled into complex chains and aggregated in lipoprotein structures called chylomicrons, consisting of triglycerides, phospholipids, cholesterol and proteins. Chylomicrons, which being water-soluble allow the transport of lipids in aqueous media, come out of the cells and are harvested in the lymph vessels. The so-enriched lymph has a milky appearance, called *chyle*, and will bring chylomicrons up to the subclavian vein, where the lymphatic bed converges into the bloodstream, which from this moment will take care of everything up to the liver.

What remains of intestinal contents continues the path to the large intestine. Also divided into several sections: *cecum*, with its small vermiform appendage belonging to the immune system, *ascending colon, transverse colon* and *descending colon*. It secretes only mucus, necessary to facilitate the passage of the contents and has as main function the absorption of water, up to seven liters per day. This function is essential for the maintenance and control of the homeostatic equilibrium of the organism.

At this point it would be appropriate to write something on the bacterial flora that lives permanently our digestive system, with greater concentration and variety in the colon. But it is dedicated to the chapter that follows, and here only mention its most important functions: the breakdown of substances that our system is not able to digest, such as cartilage and cellulose, or the synthesis of other substances to us indispensable like vitamin K, essential in blood clotting.

We have come to the end of the journey, it remains to eliminate the waste material, now transformed into stools, through the rectum.

The mechanism of digestion proved to be complex but incredibly efficient. It is important to emphasize that the choice of ingested foods is essential to keep all gears in perfect function. A diet that is too heavy and unbalanced, too fat, too rich in protein or refined starches, all of which compromises its functioning. Every day we can hear our friends' complaints, ulcer, constipation, meteorism (tympanites), diarrhea, these are the most common diseases, but also the terrible colon cancer, which hits more and more frequently. These diseases in the digestive system are caused by ourselves. By the lack of attention and respect for our body.

This book is intended to give all its readers the basics in order to fully understand the meaning that this respect must have to ensure a healthy and happy life for all of us.

Because no one of us can say more: "*I didn't know*".

9 THE BACTERIAL FLORA

In Biology, the generic term used to define coexistence between organisms of different species, animals or plants, is Symbiosis (from Greek sumbiōsis, συμβίωσις, sum "with" + bios "life"). Depending on the type of relationship between organisms, called symbionts, there are several modes of symbiosis: mutualism, when there is mutual benefit; commensalism, when the two bodies have a common use of food resources with the sole benefit of one, without, however, harming each other; Inquiline, when one of the two lives on or inside the other, or it occupies the hole, but without causing damage; finally, parasitism, the most disgusting condition. In which the advantage of one of the symbionts corresponds to a disadvantage of the other.

Perhaps the most important and underestimated mutual symbiosis we are aware of is what exists between us and the bacterial flora that inhabits our bodies.

At this point, an important point needs to be clarified. The term flora, of common use, is inaccurate or incorrect. It is reported to the vegetable world to which the bacteria were mistakenly inscribed in the past. In our day the correct term is gut microbiota or gastrointestinal microbiota. In particular, the human gut microbiota includes all the bacteria, and not only, that inhabit our organism. Gastrointestinal microbiota, means all bacteria living in the digestive tract.

According to recent studies, between 500 and 1000 different species of microorganisms inhabit the human body, the vast majority of which are anaerobic bacteria. Of these, the major group lives in the digestive tube, with a strong propensity for the colon, just know that 60% of the stomach mass is formed by bacteria.

An organ in the organ, so you can define the billions of bacteria that live in our digestive system. A "ghost" organ of vital importance. Its role is through the inhibition of pathogenic microorganisms, stimulation of the immune system, synthesis of vitamins and the improvement of the biological functions in general and in particular digestive systems. In fact, it is able to demolish molecules, such as cellulose, on which our digestive system is incapable of acting.

A different organ for each individual, because each one of us has his own microbial. It develops in the newborn baby immediately after delivery (as it is until then the gastro-intestinal tube completely sterile) due to contact with the mother's facial and reproductive apparatus as well as through breastfeeding. Within a month it reaches full maturation. In the case of caesarean delivery or nutrition based on breast milk substitutes it takes almost six months before the intestinal flora (for simplicity I will continue to refer to it in these terms) comes to its maximum efficiency. It is important to know that during this time the baby may be subject to a deficiency of vitamin K, normally synthesized by these bacteria and necessary for proper blood clotting. Modern medicine, always ready to give little confidence to natural human development, the result of millions of years of evolution, prescribes synthetic vitamin K injections at this time.

These two particular pathways lead to the development of two very different bacterial flora. The first, of natural origin, specific for humans, consisting mainly of *Bifidobacteria*, the second, originated from the environment and nutrition, characterized by *Enterobacteriaceae* and *Enterococcus*. This also happens in the case of prolonged antibiotic treatment. Antibiotics, taken in order to cure from a bacterial infection, are not able to distinguish good from bad and cause complete and total destruction of the intestinal bacterial flora. Hence, the importance, during treatment, of the intake of lactic ferments for restoration, at least in part. As we have said, after a similar destruction, the flora that is reformed in the intestine is very different from the original one, not to mention that in the period between the end of the old flora and the restoration of the new one, which can last several weeks, we remain possible targets of pathogenic bacterial strains that find fertile soil to reproduce, without competition of any kind. Strains that could have an antibiotic-resistance, so extremely dangerous. It is good to be careful, in a similar situation, also to the deficiency of vitamins normally synthesized by bacteria. It is essential to take them with fruits and vegetables, certainly not with chemical supplements whose efficiency and bioavailability is almost nothing.

The bacterial species living in humans are hundreds and variables among the populations, even among individuals of the same ethnicity, being linked, in addition to the genetics of the individual, also and mainly to the different eating habits. In fact, the gut microbiota is sensitive to food that reaches the gastrointestinal tract. It can promote the development of some species on other species or species that can cause pathologies. Many bacteria, in fact, are useful and harmless, about 80% cause fermentation (lactobacillus and bifidobacteria), but the remaining 20% causes the putrefaction of the remains (*Escherichia, Bacteroides, Eubacteria, Clostridium*) and individually they can be very dangerous, sometimes deadly. The toxins they produce are the cause of diarrhea, infections, liver damage, cancer, etc. Here is one of the reasons why the balance of flora and proper nutrition are the basics of health.

To understand even better we consider the case of *Lactobacillus*. They are part of a bacterial strain that tends to acidify the environment in which it is found, preventing the proliferation of putrefactive bacteria, which, however, prefer a basic environment. In the case of slow intestinal transit and constipation, we see a collapse of their number, with rapid growth of putrefying bacteria, dating back to the intestinal tract and causing meteorism and synthesis of pathogenic amino acids such as histamine, tyramine, cadaverine, putrescine, agmatine, mercaptan and indole.

In 450 BC Hippocrates, Father of Medicine, said, "Do that food is your medicine" and "Who does not know the food can not understand human illnesses." He obviously had the clearer ideas of many contemporary men. And contemporaries, today, have finally decided to study food and nutrition according to the logic of its ancient insights. From this was born the concept of food that can promote the growth and well-being of beneficial bacteria, characteristic of the human digestive tract.

This is the prebiotic food. It stimulates the development and activity of useful intestinal microorganisms, modulates intestinal transit and fermentative activity, reduces ammonia production and controls intestinal disorders.

Ultimately, the gut microbiota, to function efficiently and in a healthy way, must be fed with prebiotic foods specific to its nature: *fibers* (cellulose, hemicellulose, pectin, gums, lignin), *polyunsaturated fatty acids* (vegetable oils of flaxseed, pumpkin, sunflower, olive), *omega 3 fatty acids* (vegetable oils, nuts and legumes), *carotenoids* and vitamin *A*, lutein (spinach, broccoli, peas, lettuce, parsley), *lycopene* (tomato, grapefruit, mango, watermelon), *zeaxanthin* (yellow-orange vegetables, dark green vegetables), *beta-carotene* (carrots, pumpkin, peppers, apricots), *polyphenols, flavonoids* (olives, onion, garlic, cabbage, lettuce, blueberry, tomatoes, apples, apricots), *isoflavones* (soybeans and legumes), *anthocyanins* (red fruits, grapes, red oranges)). The list is long and complex, but I would like to point out that it does not include any kind of animal food: no meat, no dairy products, no fish. Foods, on the other hand, that favor the growth and development of putrefying bacterial strains, certainly not friends of life.

Many researchers agree on the ability of the gut microbiota to release hormones in the bloodstream, targeting some organs of the central nervous system, which can alter our character and our mood.

Once again, the diet becomes the key to our well-being. If through the intake of proper foods our gut microbiota will be healthy and happy, we will be healthy and happy too. The symbiotic relationship, after all, is just that.

10 CIRCADIAN RHYTHMS

The Milky Way owes its name to the look it has, seen from Earth, a bright street paved with stars. Actually, its shape is quite different. In fact, our galaxy has what is called a flattened spiral shape with a swollen center whose denseness of stars gives an incredible brightness. All the stars belonging to the Milky Way run around the core and our beloved Sun does not escape the rule. It, which lies at the edge of the spiral, has a period of revolution of about 40,000 years. Earth, the third planet of the solar system, starting from its center, turns around its star in about 365 days. During this period, an elliptical orbit takes it to approach or move away from the Sun. In addition, having our planet an inclined axis of rotation, we notice a change in the inclination of the solar rays on its surface and in the length of the day / night cycle. All this causes the change of seasons. As mentioned, the earth also makes a rotation around itself in about 24 hours.

Our satellite, the Moon, travels around the Earth in about 28 days, always keeping the same face on our planet. The gravitational attraction of the Sun, the Moon and, to a minimum, the other planets of our solar system, determine the tidal motions that macroscopically affect the oceans and seas and, less clearly, on the continental land.

Already in a distant past, ancient peoples such as the Mayans, for example, understood that all these motions, all these revolutions, could be summarized in a calendar. The attempt to describe in a schematic and mathematical manner the nature surrounding us. To harness the seasons, the ages, in order to understand the changes and to find an order that would help to deal with life. The Mayan calendar is still a marvel of the human intellect, something incredible, given the age and the technological degree of the people who created it.

Why all this talk? To introduce an important feature of the cosmos, the *cyclical nature of many events*. A feature with which life on Earth has had to face since its inception. The day and night cycles, the seasons, with temperature changes and the length of the days, tidal movements and moon phases. All this has influenced the development and evolution of life. It is a huge planetary clock, a perfect mechanism that works for billions of years, scanning seconds, minutes, hours, days, months, years, centuries, eons.

At this point we are ready to introduce a new concept, Chronobiology. The study of the times of life, that is, of the periodic changes of the vital processes of every living being. In short, the biorhythm study.

Terrestrial life forms have evolved following and adapting to the natural cycles of our planet. From the smallest prokaryotic cell to the most complex life forms to us, all of our chemical reactions, our vital processes, follow these biological rhythms. It is so deeply rooted in us that time cycles are no longer simply linked to external conditions, such as light and darkness, but are deeply tied to our DNA, transmitted by our fathers. Here, then, we find daily cycles even in people who, for study purposes, have remained in an isolated natural environment, even in the presence of changing environmental parameters such as days and nights altered in their length.

Biological cycles are normally divided according to their duration: *ultradiane*, when they range from 1 millisecond to a few hours, for example breathing, heartbeat, or the sense of hunger that reappear after a few hours; *circadian*, when they have a period of about one day, sleep and wake; *infradian*, when they have a period of one week, one month or one year, as the menstrual cycle or, in specific season, allergic rhinitis and some forms of depression.

Of particular interest in modern medicine are the cycles that regulate human hormone metabolism. The subject is very complex and is out of this discussion. However, it is useful to know that the most important hormone concentration is linked to night / day cycles, and although some of them last for twenty-four hours, we see peaks in some phase of the day.

Daily cycles are the ones most interested in feeding study.

The term circadian comes from Latin *circa diem*, "about a day", and was coined by researcher Franz Halberg around 1950. Daily cycles were known and studied, however, since antiquity and was around 1729 that the French scholar Jean-Jacques d'Ortous de Mairan understood that biological cycles were of endogenous origin, that is, of biological metabolism and not simply induced by environmental changes.

In fact, he observed that plant movements, linked to the light / dark cycle, actually continued even when the plant was subjected to constant darkness. These remarks pave the way for a new way of studying the subject, which led to modern theory. The ever-expanding study has continued to this day, allowing us to explain cyclical processes in a very precise and accurate way. Let's take for example the light / dark cycle. Its origin is certainly of the oldest, it is traced back to the first protocells appearing on Earth.

They, which were the first forms of vegetable life to attempt to colonize the emerged lands, had the need to protect the replication of DNA from ultraviolet radiation, which due to the different atmospheric composition was not sufficiently screened. For this reason replication was done at night. We find today in the *Neurospora* fungus this control mechanism.

As organic matter evolves and life complexity is increased, even circadian rhythmic regulation increases enormously in complexity. To better understand, we make the example of the synthesis of the *melatonin* hormone. It is secreted by the *pineal gland*. The target organ on which it exercises the greatest control is the *suprachiasmatic nucleus*, organ of the very active central nervous system, in turn controlling sleep and wake mechanisms. Melatonin, therefore, indirectly, is the hormone best suited to regulating sleep and wake states. Precisely its function makes the circadian rhythm so important, to which itself is strictly subjected. In fact, the hormone is secreted only at night.

The synthesis begins shortly after the appearance of darkness, blood concentration tends to increase rapidly with peaks between 2 and 4 a.m., then decelerate when approaching the morning. Thanks to the action of the photoreceptors present on the eye retina, the ambient light stimuli produce an increase in secretion in the presence of darkness and an inhibition in the presence of light.

It is interesting to note that, in individuals who voluntarily underwent isolation from natural conditions, sleep / wake rhythm slowly shifted over 36 hours rather than 24 correct ones. This phenomenon is very important to understand that although the circadian clock is endogenous, that is, of the body itself and programmed directly into DNA, environmental stimuli still have a role of regulation and synchronization with the world around us.

Finally, the function of melatonin in the control of the immune system and secretion of pancreatic hormones, such as insulin and glucagon, has been proven; and, again, in strengthening the lowering mechanism of the nocturnal body temperature through the vasodilatation of the peripheral circulatory system, to facilitate the propensity to sleep.

As usual, the biological mechanisms of our body prove to be linked and interconnected among themselves in the most unexpected way. The overturning of the sleep / wake cycle affects our ability to defend us from external illnesses and agents, compromises blood glucose balance and as we shall see, it will soon be reflected in our entire well-being. Still a word: according to recent statistics, internet night-use is changing the habits of the population, with a significant decrease in the hours of sleep. You are left to make up your own mind.

Worldwide medical-hygienist literature is rich in treaties aimed at seeking a link between circadian or biological rhythms in general and healthy eating.

Most researchers agree to establish in three main cyclical stages human food metabolism: the first phase, called the *Appropriation cycle* (food intake and digestion), from noon to 8 pm; the second phase, which takes the name of *Assimilation cycle* (absorption and management of nutrients ingested in the first phase) from 8 pm to 4 am; and finally, the third stage, called *Elimination* (which, as its name suggests, deals with the elimination of waste and toxins accumulated in the body during the day) runs from 4 am to noon.

It is very important to respect these three phases. Interrupt or compromise one of the three phases during their development unbalances all the biological equilibrium of our body.

This is a very controversial topic, classical food science does not agree generally with this theory, although in recent years the number of doctors who are approaching it, challenging what canonical methodologies are, is growing more and more.

But what do in practical these phases mean and what are the habits we have to do to respect them?

As we saw the elimination phase starts at 4 am and continues until noon. If we do an abundant breakfast in the morning, we force the body to move energy resources to the digestive system for digestion, subtracting them from the operations necessary to perform properly the stage, perhaps the most important of the three, because it takes care of taking off the body toxins and metabolism residues accumulated during the day. If we stop this phase we does not allow the body to clean itself up and compromise its regenerative capacity. As we will see in the chapter on excretory organs, the repercussions at physiological level are enormous. At this point it is important to know that fasting is not necessary, but it is important to ingest only foods with a zero digestive impact, that means, fruit. Only it, thanks to the presence of self-healing enzymes, will be accepted by the body without compromising any phase.

At this point, continuing to follow the logic of the three phases every day, it is clear that meals should be made during the appropriation phase. It is important, however, to know that they do not have to be excessive, but I think this is clear to everyone. The digestion of a heavy and too abundant meal is, in fact, prolonged over time and requires an excessive amount of energy in the body. Especially in the evening, it is important to dine early, at least three hours before the start of the assimilation phase. In fact, if digestion is still ongoing, there is a slowdown and a delay in this second phase. This will affect the body's ability to absorb and manage the nutritious elements taken during meals. Everything is balance, every moment of the three phases is important, metabolic deficiencies, overweight, obesity and many diseases, all linked together with a thin wire that is very easy to break.

The cycles as we have seen are quite stiff and each one requires its time, so a too heavy dinner, whose digestion extends throughout the night, will in the end also compromise the third stage, that of elimination, in a vicious cycle that is prolonged in time, unbalancing the equilibrium for several days.

Balances that affect our health, the immune system, the endocrine system, the excretory system, the circulatory system and the nervous system.

Everything is interconnected.

11 THE FOUR
CHANNELS OF ELIMINATION

Excretory Organs

Like many men I deeply love the sea. An endless stretch of water, always in motion, rich in life and capable of giving us amazing landscapes. Perhaps my love is linked to the sense of freedom that the sea represents or perhaps this feeling is related to a memory: the ancestral memory of when our ancestors swam in it millions of years before colonizing the land.

Poetically I could say that I always carry the sea inside me and, in the end, this would be a biological truth too. Because 80% of the body's weight is made of water. 62% of all this water is located in the cells, the blood is 12% and the remaining 26% consists of the extracellular fluids which constitute the lymph.

In this incredible amount of water, all the substances in life are dissolved, all in perfect osmotic and ionic balance, all in exact concentrations so that cells that are immersed in it can live and with them we can live. And who knows some of these cells are not yet convinced to be immersed in the sea?

From a certain perspective, the environment in which we move is hostile because is dry, we have to fight a small daily war to keep water in the right amount in our body, nourish, drink, control the temperature, eliminate metabolic waste, everything must be done balancing perfectly the hydro-saline balance. The concentrations of intra and extra cellular substances must remain strictly constant. This work, already complex in a healthy individual, adds to the elimination of all the toxins that can invade our organism due to a bad diet or unhealthy habits, such as smoke and alcohol, or, again, because of environmental and climatic factors, such as atmospheric pollution or water sources.

What a wonderful machine is a living organism! During your life, have you ever considered how many complications allowed us to walk on the surface of this planet? To enjoy the beauty of our life, the love of our affections?

The skin, kidneys, lungs, colon, lymphatic system and finally the liver, these are the organs involved to carry out this highly complex control, commonly called *complex of the excretory organs*. We now realize that the elimination of substances is only a small part of their task.

Organs for excellence of the excretory system are *kidneys, urinary tract, bladder*.

The kidneys

The kidneys are two, with the characteristic bean shape, with the internal curvature turned towards the center of the body, from which the urinate cavities go out and then continue to the bladder, in which they discharge the produced urine. The kidney functions are essential for life: the so-called kidney block causes the individual to die in 3/4 days. They are: filtering and elimination from blood of toxic or waste substances, control of osmotic and ionic concentrations, resulting in adjustment of pH, control the amount of water circulating in the body.

The *nefrone* is the functional unit of the kidney. It consists of two distinct sections, the renal *glomerulus* and kidney *tubule*. The first is formed by a set of small convoluted canals in close contact with the blood capillaries that sprout abundantly the organ; the contact surface has microscopic pores from which pass part of the serum and the smallest molecules, below the effect of blood pressure. It's a real mechanical filter. The second is born from the glomerulus and it is a U shape tubule of a slightly thicker section, whose function is to convey the liquid filtered (which takes the name of *pre-urine*), towards the urinary passages that will then take it up to the bladder. Usually eliminated substances are urea, uric acid, ammonia, salicylic acid, purine, xanthine, ptomaine and salts, that is, waste products of metabolism.

Each day, about 1700 liters of pre-urine are filtered through the glomerulus, it is clear that such a watery mole needs to be reabsorbed in some way and this is exactly what the kidney tubules deal with.

Their surface is littered with active pump systems, which, selectively carrying ions from side to side of the tubular membrane, operate the resorption of the water contained in the pre-urine against the gradient of pressure and concentration. All this requires a lot of work for the kidney and a great expense of energy. With the water, others substances are recovered, that have been able to pass the filter but that are still needed. All this work, besides allowing us to preserve the right volume of body fluids, also allows to adjust the pH of the blood. In fact, it is at this level that by controlling the passage of acid ions or bases, the kidney contributes substantially to maintaining the value at around 7.41 (very similar to that of sea water!). But it's still not enough. Like all organs of our body, the kidney also has many functions. It is the case that we, by eating, do not know the concentrations of nutrients we enter into our body. But life needs defined values and clear balances for each substance; It is clear, therefore, that the control of the nutrient concentrations of the kidney is of fundamental importance to it. By eliminating in surplus substances, but by holding those whose concentration is lower than the due, it ensures the right nutrient supply to our cells.

We now understand that the man machine is very complex and that its organs often have many functions. Another example is the skin.

The skin

The epidermis completely covers our body. In addition to the actual containment function, it has a lot of other assignments. *Thermoregulation*: by sweating, controlling and maintaining body temperature, at this level, by opening and closing the myriad of pores disseminated on its surface, it participates in the mechanism of fever. Protection from *mechanical agents*, such as solar radiation, due to melanin synthesis, or impacts against objects; by *chemical agents*, for example, urticating substances and, finally, by *biological agents*: the hydrolipidic film that renders it makes it impermeable to the attacks of microorganisms. But beware, the skin is not waterproof to everything, many chemicals actually penetrate and through this, reach the bloodstream that spray it abundantly. These substances can be drugs, see new skin patches for heart or travel illness, or potentially toxic poisons, such as clothing dyes, perfumes, and metals such as lead, for example.

The problem is that the absorption through the skin has a very high efficiency, there is not, in fact, the first-pass effect that we discussed in the chapter on the liver. This is considered an advantage by pharmacists (less active substance is needed to achieve the desired result) but it is a danger to our health, just a low concentration of poison to get devastating effects. The toxic agent, in fact, must not overcome the obstruction of the liver before reaching the target organs and spreading throughout the body.

Skin, through a myriad of sensors, *proprioceptors* (pain sensors), *thermoreceptors*, *pressoreceptors* and others, allows us to interface with the world around us.

What would our life be without touch?

Last but not least, the skin is part of the group of the excretory organs.

It is, in fact, the means by which numerous chemicals pass through, accumulating in the blood due to the fatigue of the internal organs.

Eczema and boils, bad smell, they are typical symptoms of an inner malaise of our body and attempts by it to eliminate toxins that are accumulating. It is obvious at this point that treating these so-called skin diseases with creams is quite useless, but they can alleviate the nuisances caused by the symptoms, but first of all we need to cure the inside of the body and bring back the right balance.

At that point the skin will return bright and soft, completely healed.

The lungs

It's time to take a good breath, breathe deeply, wait a few seconds and then exhale, exhale again, here, you feel better.

In recent years, respiratory diseases have hit more and more people and at an ever lower age. The incidence in large cities is reaching very high limits, almost all the inhabitants. Allergies, colds, tonsillitis, various inflammations, atmospheric pollution is certainly among the major causes, but it is not the only guilty, we will see why now.

The respiratory apparatus involves a large number of organs, some in common with other apparatus, such as the immune system and the excretory system.

Nose, mouth, larynx and pharynx, trachea, bronchi and, finally, lungs: all enrolled in breathing.

For this treatment we will not dwell on the upper tract, but we will only examine trachea, bronchi and lungs.

The lungs are two, contained and protected from the rib cage. The upper conical extremities arrive until they slip between the clavicle and the scapula, and at the bottom they end with the base put on the diaphragm; they are both wrapped in a double membrane, called *pleura*, which allows them to be fixed to the rib cage. The left lung is slightly smaller than the right for the presence of the heart.

The trachea, descending, divides into two bronchi, after passing through the neck. These are then branched into ever smaller branches penetrating into their own lungs, which become bronchioles and reach microscopic dimensions, finally ending in the pulmonary alveoli, the actual functional unit. The pulmonary artery coming from the right ventricle of the heart is divided into two branches that, following the bronchi in their path, are divided into so many branches by penetrating the lung parenchyma and ending in capillaries that envelop the alveoli; from these capillaries then oxygen-enriched blood is harvested in ever larger vessels until they get out of the lungs. It then takes the road to the right atrium of the heart in the pulmonary vein and closes the small circulation.

Don't be annoyed for this boring disquisition, because we have to clear the complication, but also the great efficiency of the man machine. So again, we build a chain of events: during breathing the diaphragm lowers and the chest muscles enlarge the volume of the rib cage. Through the pleura this movement is transmitted to the lungs which thus increase in volume. The pulmonary alveoli dilate and the fresh air coming from the upper respiratory tract penetrates in them rich in oxygen. The very fine and particularly permeable membrane that connects the alveolus with the blood capillary allows at this point the exchange of gas with the blood. Then the mechanism is reversed, the diaphragm rises, and the chest muscles compress the rib cage by exerting pressure on the compressing lungs and thus the exhalation of the air rich in carbon dioxide begins.

Hemoglobin, contained in red blood cells, is a complex molecule with a group called *heme*, in which we find an iron atom. In the presence of a high concentration of O2, the heme group, with a fairly complex set of reactions, releases carbon dioxide molecules from the venous circulation and captures oxygen to distribute it throughout the body. It is necessary to know that the group, once reached the periphery, is immersed in a poorly oxygenated but rich carbon dioxide environment and this causes the reaction to reverse with oxygen release and transport of carbon dioxide to the lungs. The reactions related to the transport of carbon dioxide occur on the basis of mechanisms that can change the pH.

This is one of the reasons why breathing is one of the body's systems to adjust your pH. In the presence of an acid pH, certain sensors scattered around the body control the increase in respiratory rate and this brings the values to the right level. Here it becomes clear how good breathing control and good oxygenation are so important to health.

The trachea and bronchi are covered by a mucosa rich in cells that emit a particular viscous and sticky mucus. In addition, the entire surface has vibrating lashes which, by their movement, generate a flow that leads the mucus upward to pour into the esophagus. This is a very important function: the incoming air is rich in microorganisms, dust particles and pollutants, the air swirler makes sure that all of this goes to slam and remains trapped in the mucus and then digested. Smoking damages lashes that interrupt their movement, mucus tends to stagnate in the bronchi and this gives the characteristic and so annoying phlegm cough of chronic smokers.

Why did we decide to talk about the lungs regarding the excretory system? In the presence of particularly high blood toxaemia, the kidneys and the liver struggle to eliminate the waste materials and toxins. In such a situation, which is linked to chronic illness, bad nutrition or alcoholism, the body is forced to find alternative ways for elimination. And the lung, thanks to the large permeability of the alveolar walls, is able to intervene. Waste materials accumulate in the interstices between the alveoli, to be gradually eliminated, through the respiration and through a large amount of mucus. A typical example is the tremendous breath of the alcoholics, whose damaged liver is no longer able to function properly. In these situations we are faced with a clogging of the respiratory tract with the blockage of part of the lungs literally drowned by the mucus.

This leads to the persistence of a condition that can quickly become pathological, inflammation of the pulmonary parenchyma or of the pleura, which I remember being the double membrane that surrounds the lung.

This inflammation, called pleurisy, involves the accumulation of fluid full of toxins in the space between the two membrane leaves, resulting in reduced volume to the lung itself and loss of complete respiratory capacity.

The decrease in respiratory capacity also has a secondary rather serious consequence besides the deprivation of a good air exchange. This is the inefficient control of blood pH by breathing CO_2. This results in an increase in blood acidity. It is a vicious circle, because the decrease in pH leads to an increase in work by the already suffering kidney and, in the event of its inefficiency, a buffer mechanism is introduced which removes calcium from the bones to the extreme result of assisting in the onset of osteoporosis.

Everything is tied up in the body, balance, stability, equilibrium. I never tire of writing it.

The lymphatic system, which we discussed in the chapter dedicated to the immune system, collect the *lymph*, a clear liquid similar to blood serum, which fills all the extracellular spaces. It is not, as in the case of the circulatory system, a closed circle.

Out of the extracellular spaces, the lymph drains into very small ducts that connect from the periphery to each other, running inside the muscles and becoming bigger until they reach the lymphatic vessel which runs from the abdomen to the chest and pours into the vena cava right into the circulatory blood bed.

The lymphatic system does not have a real propulsion organ but is subject to the continuous pressures generated by the muscles in which it flows, the presence of numerous non-return valves forces the lymphatic flow to go into a single direction, avoiding reflux. Throughout the path of lymph vessels, particularly in the vicinity of the main organs or blood vessels, lymphatic stations are present, called lymph nodes.

In the lymph nodes, there is a great concentration of B and T *lymphocytes*, the immune system's stations which handle with the control of immune reaction. At the level of the high respiratory tract, larynx and pharynx, we find other developed lymph nodes called *tonsils*, which in addition to being sensors capable of detecting the presence of pathogenic microorganisms, to trigger an immediate immune reaction, are able to expel toxins present in amount in the lymph, collected at extracellular spaces throughout the body.

The intestine

The last tract of the intestine, the *colon*, is also the last organ we will deal with within this chapter. Unfortunately, however, for my need for completeness, we must first try to locate and understand this organ of vital importance.

The intestine is the terminal part of the digestive system; it reaches an average of 7 meters in length, it is divided into several parts, all with specific tasks. The first part, the longest, is the small intestine, divided into three parts, duodenum, jejunum and ileum, a long soft tissue tube curled up on itself several times, positioned in the abdomen, between the stomach and the large intestine. In it through the pancreatic juices, bile salts, duodenal enzymes and particular bacteria, digestion of amino acids, amides and fatty acids occurs. The small intestine ends in the cecum, the first part of the large intestine. From this continues in the three sections of the colon, ascending, transversal and descending, to end in the rectum that end up into the anus. The large intestine has essentially the task of re-absorbing the remaining digestion fluids, between 900 and 1400 ml per day.

I recall the importance of the bacterial flora that lives in our gut, which we have already talked about, that takes care of digesting some substances, synthesizing vitamins and fighting the pathogenic flora and toxins that it produces.

The importance of the intestine, and in particular of the *colon*, in the elimination of waste and residues of digestion, as well as toxins, is now clear.

As it also appears clear the importance of keeping the organ absolutely in order. A diet based on animal products, poor in plant fibers, causes intestinal laziness and constipation. This involves feces stagnation for too long, with advanced putrefactive phenomena, release of toxic substances, including carcinogens and blockage of functionalities.

The intestinal wall is a passage for substances rejection of our body, once again, when the excretory organs are fatigued, the body looks for new ways to eliminate toxins and the colon is just one of these means. But if it is clogged because of a diet of animal proteins and refined starches that make glues, such as non-integral white flour or rice, this path is blocked.

In addition, since the intestinal walls are highly permeable to liquids and substances (it is true that the parenteral route has been used for many years for drug intake, such as suppositories... no first-pass effect, remember?), intestine clogging increases alarmingly the vein load against which the organism will have to fight. It is interesting to know that there are numerous studies that have shown the statistical correlation between a diet rich in animal proteins and refined starches and colon cancer, which hits every year a slice of ever-larger population. The same studies show that a diet rich in vegetable fibers can reverse the trend, just taking at least 10 grams of fiber per day to reduce the risk percentage by more than 40 percent.

At this point we can draw conclusions: all the organs of a healthy body have specific functions for which they have evolved over the millennia. In the man machine, however, there are redundant systems able to provide and overcome the inefficiency of an organ, replacing at least partially its functions for short periods.

A healthy, balanced diet rich in fruits and vegetables, possibly raw, keeps all the organs in perfect efficiency, the body is in balance with itself and with the world in which it moves.

Unfortunately, our society constantly target us with poisons, toxic substances, garbage, animal food, dairy products and more, forcing our organs to continue an endless ride to the pursuit of that balance, with the result that extra work compromises their functionality, forces them to assume roles for which they are not designed, consuming them daily more and more.

It is a vicious circle: a compromised balance affects others, in a cascading effect that makes us sick, weak, nervous, susceptible and aggressive.

Is this really what we want to be?

Keep reading...
You can find out more about CORRECT NUTRITION
in my next book: *"How to find health - Step 2"*
Click here now: https://goo.gl/yQbj1E

"Tell The World What You Think Of This Book.
Would you mind taking a few seconds
to leave an honest review?
It's important because your opinion
helps people make better decisions."

Diego Pagani

Author	Title	Year	Edition
Ehret, Arnold	*Prof. Arnold Ehret's Mucusless Diet Healing System*	1924	Ehret Literature
Peter Jentschura	la salute attraverso eliminazione delle scorie	2006	Jentschura Verlag
Harvey e Marlin Diamond	A tutta salute	1989	Sperling & Kupfer S.p.A.
A.M. King	io sono immortale	2010	Io sono Edizioni
4	la vita segreta delle piante		
Max Gerson	Gerson Therapy Handbook	1999	Gerson Institute
Edmond Bordeaux Szekely	il vangelo esseno	2006	manca edizioni
norman walker	Succhi Freschi di Frutta e Verdura	2012	Macro edizioni
Deepak Chopra	Corpo senza eta mente senza tempo	2005	Sperling & Kupfer S.p.A.
Herbert M. Shelton	il digiuno puo salvarvi la vita	1986	Società Editrice Igiene Naturale s.r.l.
William Dufty	Sugar Blues	2005	Macro edizioni

T. Colin Campbell	The China study	2011	Macro edizioni
Anatomia Umana	Paolo Castano, Lucio Cocco, Alessandra De Barbieri, Loredana D'Este, Francesca Floriani, Gherardo Gheri, Maria Rita Mondello, Stefano Papa, Pietro Petriglieri, Giuliano Pizzini, Carlo Ridola, Stelio Rossi, Giovanni Sacchi, Paola Sirigu, Salvatore Spinella	2003	edi-ermes
Renzo Minelli	Appunti di fisiologia umana. Programma per la tabella XVIII, fisiologia della respirazione e dell'equilibrio acido base	2013	Editore Medea
B. B. Buchanan	Biochimica e biologia molecolare delle piante	2003	Zanichelli
Reginald H. Garrett	Reginald H. Garrett	2008	Zanichelli
Graham Hancock	Impronte degli dei	1992	TEA
Graham Hancock	Talismano. Le città sacre e la Fede segreta	2004	TEA
Henry Gray	Anatomy of the human body	1918	*Lea & Febiger*
Frank H. Netter,	*Atlante di anatomia umana, 3ª edizione*	2007	*Elsevier Masson*

Zaccaria Fumagalli	*Anatomia umana normale*	1983	Piccin
Dee Unglaub Silverthorn	*Fisiologia umana*	2010	*Pearson Education Italia*
Luigi Grazioli, Lucio Olivetti	*Diagnostica per immagini delle malattie del fegato e delle vie biliari*	2005	*Elsevier*
Charles A. Janeway, Paul Travers, Mark Walport, Mark J. Shlomchik	*Immunobiologia (3ª edizione italiana sulla 6ª inglese)*	2007	Piccin
Giuliano Ricciotti	*Biochimica di base*	2008	*Italo Bovolenta*
V. Donald, Voet Judith G. e Pratt Charlotte W	*Fondamenti di biochimica,*	2001	Zanichelli
Berg Jeremy M., Tymoczko John L. e Stryer Lubert	*Biochimica*	2003	Zanichelli
H. J. M. Bowen	*Trace Flements in Biochemistry*	1976	Academic Press
Carlo M. Rotella, Edoardo Mannucci, Barbara Cresci	*Criteri diagnostici e terapia*	1999	*SEE Editrice Firenze*
Giovanni Faglia, Paolo Beck-Peccoz	*del sistema endocrino e del metabolismo 4ª edizione*	2006	*McGraw-Hill*

Research Laboratories Merck	*Merck Manual quinta edizione*	2008	*Springer-Verlag*
Gremigni P, Letizia L	*Il problema obesità. Manuale per tutti i professionisti della salute*	2011	*Maggioli Editore*
William E. Winter, Maria Rita Signorino, Diabetes Mellitus	*Pathophysiology, Etiologies, Complications, Management, and Laboratory Evaluation*	####	*Assoc. for Clinical Chemistry*
Fumento, Michael	*The Fat of the Land: Our Health Crises and How Overweight Americans can Help Themselves*	1997	*Penguin Books*
Keller, Kathleen	Encyclopedia of Obesity	2008	*Sage Publications, Inc*
Kolata, Gina, Rethinking Thin	*new science of weight loss - and the myths and realities of dieting*	2007	Picador
Levy-Navarro, Elena	*The Culture of Obesity in Early and Late Modernity*	2008	*Palgrave Macmillan*
) Pool, Robert, Fat	*Fighting the Obesity Epidemic*	2001	*Oxford, UK*
M. Wabitsch, J. Hebebrand, W. Kiess, K. Zwiauer	*Child and Adolescent Obesity: Causes and Consequences, Prevention and Management*	2004	*Springer*

M. Wabitsch, J. Hebebrand, W. Kiess, K. Zwiauer	*Child and Adolescent Obesity*	2005	Piper
Manzi G	*L'evoluzione umana. Ominidi e uomini prima di Homo sapiens*	2007	Il Mulino
Hermann Bengtson	Introduction to Ancient History	1975	University of California Press
Hulda Regehr Clark	The Cure for All Cancers	1993	New Century Press
Alex Jack	Il cibo medicina	2005	Hermes
Bates Williams	Vista perfetta senza occhiali - ebook	2014	Loredana de Michelis
Wilson Lawrence	Equilibrio nutrizionale e analisi minerale tessutale		Sinai Edizioni
Rothwell NJ, Stock MJ	Influence of carbohydrate and fat intake on diet-inuduced thermobenesis and brown fat activity	1987	J Nutr 117
Stirling Jl, Stock MJ	Metabolic originis of thermogenesis by diet	1968	nature 200
Horio F, Youngman LD, Bell RC	Thermogenesis, low-protein diets and decresed development of AFB1-induced preneoplastic foci in rat liver	1991	Nutr Cancer 16

Youngman LD	The growth and development of aflatoxin B1-induced preneoplastic lesion, tumors, metastasis and spontaneous tumors as they are influence by dietary protein level.	1990	Ph.D Thesis 1990
Robbins J.	The food Revolution	2001	Barkeky, CA
Macilwain G.	The general nature and treatment of Tumors	1845	John Churchill
Associated press	Survey: many guidelines qritten by doctor with ties to companies	2002	The Itaca Journal 12 Feb
Olivieri NF	Patients' health or company profits? The commercialization of academy reserch.	2003	Engineering Ethics
Chopra SS	Industry funding of clinical trials: benefect or bias?	2003	Jama 290
Moyniham R.	Who pays dor the pizza? Redefining the relationships between doctor and drug company	2003	Brit. Med. Journal 326
Eberhardt MV, Lee CY, Liu RH	Antioxidant activity of fresh apples	2000	Nature 405
Boseley S.	Sugar industry threatens to scupper WHO	2003	The Guardian 21 April

Author	Title	Year	Publisher
Albert CM, Hennekens CH, O'Donnell CJ	Fish consumption and risk of sudden cardiac death	1998	Jama 289
Informatio Plus	Nutrition a key to good health	1999	information Plus
Valdo Vaccaro	Alimentazione Naturale - Vol. 2 - Libro	2014	Anima Edizioni
Valdo Vaccaro	Alimentazione Naturale - Vol.1- Libro	2009	Anima Edizioni
Giovannucci E, Rimm E Liu Y	A prospective study of tomato product, lycopene and prostate cancer risk	2002	Nat. Cancer Institute
Yaukey J	Changing cows diests elevates milks' caner.fighting	1996	Ithaca Journal
Joel Fuhrman	Eat to Live: The Amazing Nutrient-Rich Program for Fast and Sustained Weight Loss, Revised Edition	2011	Little brown and company
Lorenzo Acerra	Il Mal di Latte Il Mal di Latte Intolleranze,allergie e malattie da latte e latticini	2008	Macro Edizioni
Frank A. Oski	Don't Drink Your Milk!	1992	Teach Services Inc
Matthew D. Warner	Fruitarians Are The Future	2012	Independent Publishing Platform

Douglas N. Graham	The 80/10/10 Diet	2006	FoodnSport Press
Jesse J Jacoby	The Raw Cure: Healing Beyond Medicine: How self-empowerment, a raw vegan diet, and change of lifestyle can free us from sickness and disease	2012	SoulSpire
Ralph E Phd Carson	Harnessing The Healing Power Of Fruit: The New Paradigm for Optimum Health	2009	Siloam
Anne Osborne	Fruitarianism : The Path To Paradise	2009	Anne Osborne; Third Printing
Robert S. Morse N.D	The Detox Miracle Sourcebook: Raw Food and Herbs for Complete Cellular Regeneration	2004	Kalindi Press
norman walker	la salute dell'intestino	2012	Macro edizioni
Herbert M. Shelton	Food Combining Made Easy	2012	Book Pub Company; 3rd edition
Herbert M. Shelton	The History of Natural Hygiene and Principles of Natural Hygiene	2010	Kessinger Publishing, LLC
Keith Woodford	Devil in the Milk: Illness, Health and the Politics of A1 and A2 Milk	2009	Chelsea Green Publishing

"How to find health" serie:

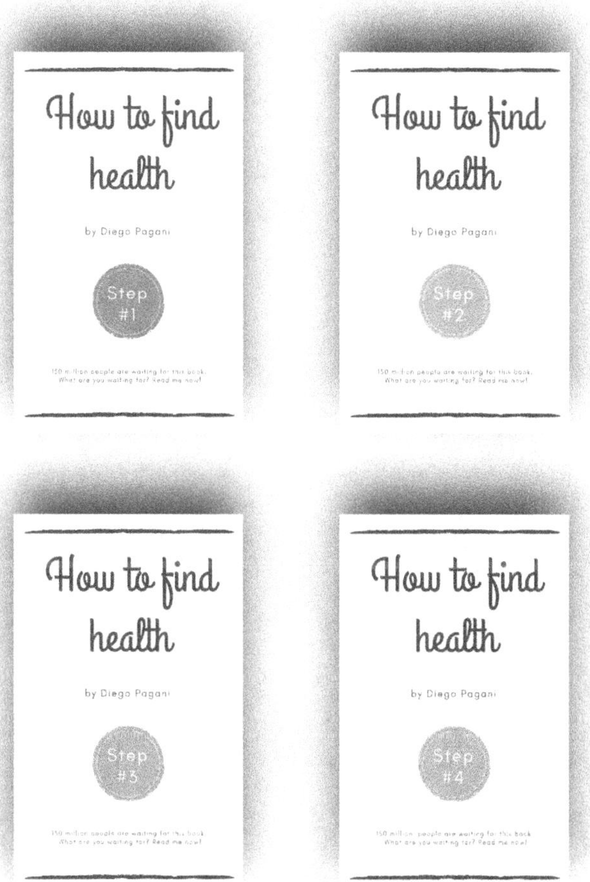

www.howfindhealth.com